THE LOST ART OF ORAL HEALING

Ancient Natural Remedies to Heal Your Mouth, Balance Your Microbiome, and Support Whole-Body Health with Modern Understanding

The Hidden Architecture

Healing begins when we remember that the mouth is not separate from the body but the doorway to its deepest balance.

Table of Contents

Introduction: Rediscovering the Forgotten Wisdom of Oral Healing

The Link Between Oral Health and Total Body Wellness

Most people see oral health as something limited to teeth and gums. If you have no cavities, no bleeding gums, and your smile looks good in photos, you might assume your mouth is in perfect shape. Yet science and traditional wisdom alike have shown that what happens in the mouth rarely stays in the mouth. The state of your oral tissues, saliva, and microbiome sends ripple effects throughout your entire body, influencing everything from heart health to immune function. Understanding this connection is the first step to transforming oral care from a purely cosmetic habit into a practice that supports long-term vitality.

Modern research has uncovered that the mouth acts as both a mirror and a gateway for systemic health. Dentists and physicians now recognize that many chronic conditions—cardiovascular disease, diabetes, even certain autoimmune disorders—often share inflammatory pathways with gum disease. In simple terms, if your gums are inflamed, the same biological triggers that affect them can travel through your bloodstream and reach distant organs. This is not meant to create alarm, but to highlight how integrated the human body truly is.

The Mouth as a Microbial Ecosystem

Your mouth hosts billions of bacteria, fungi, and other microorganisms. This community, known as the oral microbiome, functions much like the gut microbiome: it helps regulate digestion, supports immunity, and maintains a healthy barrier against harmful invaders. A balanced oral microbiome protects teeth by promoting remineralization and preventing acid-producing bacteria from taking over. When balance is lost—due to stress, poor diet, overuse of harsh mouthwashes, or smoking—harmful species can dominate, leading to gum inflammation and decay.

A study by Liu et al. (2012) mapped these microbial shifts in patients with periodontal disease, revealing clear patterns of imbalance that correlated with active inflammation. This type of research confirms what holistic traditions have long suspected: oral health is inseparable from overall wellbeing because it reflects what is happening deeper inside the body.

Chronic Inflammation and Systemic Effects

The link between oral disease and systemic conditions is largely driven by chronic inflammation. Gum disease, even in its mild stages, can release inflammatory markers into the bloodstream. Over time, these compounds contribute to vascular damage and metabolic stress. For example, studies have shown that individuals with untreated periodontal disease have a higher likelihood of developing atherosclerosis, a buildup of plaque inside the arteries. The same inflammatory molecules that irritate gums can worsen insulin resistance, making blood sugar harder to control in people with diabetes.

This does not mean that gum problems directly cause heart disease or diabetes on their own. Rather, they participate in a feedback loop: systemic conditions can worsen oral health, and poor oral health can aggravate systemic conditions. For someone seeking whole-body healing, this insight is crucial. Caring for the mouth is not only about preventing cavities, it is about lowering the overall inflammatory burden on the body.

Traditional Views of Oral–Body Connections

Ancient healing systems have always viewed the mouth as more than a set of teeth. In traditional Chinese medicine, the tongue is considered a map of internal organs. Ayurvedic practices like oil pulling aim to detoxify the body through the oral tissues, reflecting a belief that impurities in the mouth affect the entire system. While modern science uses different language— microbiome, immune response, systemic inflammation—the underlying principle is surprisingly aligned: oral care is whole-body care.

Recognizing this harmony between ancient and modern perspectives allows us to draw from both worlds. We can respect the cultural wisdom that inspired practices like herbal rinses while also validating them through emerging research. For example, when traditional systems recommended daily scraping of the tongue to remove toxins, they could not have known about bacterial biofilms, yet current studies confirm that tongue cleaning does indeed reduce bacterial load and improve breath quality.

Research continues to reveal new ways in which oral health acts as an indicator of overall wellness. Conditions like Alzheimer's disease, for instance, have been associated with certain bacteria commonly found in periodontal infections, suggesting that the mouth may play a role in the development or progression of neurodegenerative diseases. This does not mean brushing your teeth prevents dementia, but it highlights that chronic gum inflammation may contribute to a cascade of effects in the brain. Similarly, links have been observed between poor oral hygiene and respiratory infections; harmful oral bacteria can migrate to the lungs, especially in older adults or those with compromised immunity, increasing the risk of pneumonia.

The cardiovascular system is one of the most extensively studied areas in this connection. Inflammation from gum disease has been associated with thickening of the arterial walls and increased risk of clot formation. Researchers like Di Stefano (2022) emphasize that while oral bacteria themselves do not directly cause heart attacks, their byproducts can enter the bloodstream and contribute to vascular stress. Managing oral inflammation may therefore reduce an important risk factor for heart disease, particularly when combined with other lifestyle habits like a balanced diet and regular movement.

The gut also responds to oral health in ways that are only beginning to be fully understood. Oral bacteria swallowed daily can influence the composition of the gut microbiome, either supporting digestive health or worsening imbalances that lead to bloating, food sensitivities, or even autoimmune responses. Some studies, such as Komiya et al. (2019), have detected oral bacteria like *Fusobacterium nucleatum* in colorectal tissue, hinting at a potential role in intestinal disorders. This underscores that improving oral care is not only about protecting teeth but may also help create a healthier internal environment from the top of the digestive tract downward.

What makes these findings so valuable is not simply the scientific novelty but their practical implications. By recognizing that the mouth reflects and influences the entire body, oral care can become a central pillar of preventive health. Daily practices like gentle brushing with mineral-rich toothpaste, flossing or using interdental tools, and incorporating natural rinses support not just fresh breath but systemic balance. Diet also plays a significant role: nutrients such as vitamin D, vitamin K2, and magnesium contribute to strong enamel and resilient gums while also benefiting bones and cardiovascular health.

Equally important is the recognition that oral health is dynamic and responsive to lifestyle factors beyond brushing and diet. Chronic stress, for example, raises cortisol levels, which in turn can increase inflammation and slow healing in gum tissue. Lack of quality sleep can impair immune function, leaving the mouth more susceptible to harmful bacterial growth. These connections encourage a broader approach to care, where practices like stress management, regular physical activity, and adequate sleep become as important to oral wellness as the toothbrush itself.

For those seeking to create real change, it helps to view oral care as part of a larger healing routine rather than an isolated task. This perspective aligns with many ancestral practices where the health of the mouth was inseparable from spiritual and physical vitality. While modern routines may look different, the principle remains: the state of your mouth offers daily feedback on the state of your body. Bleeding gums, chronic bad breath, or recurring cavities are not just dental issues to fix temporarily but invitations to look deeper at nutrition, stress, and systemic inflammation.

As you explore the practices in upcoming chapters—herbal rinses, oil pulling, nutrient-dense foods, and daily routines—you will see how these methods work together to restore balance in the mouth and, by extension, in the body as a whole. The ultimate goal is not perfection or a flawless smile but harmony between oral care and whole-body wellness, allowing the mouth to serve as both a guardian and a guide on your path to better health.

The Philosophy of Healing the Mouth Naturally and Sustainably

Healing the mouth naturally begins with a shift in perspective. It requires us to move away from the mindset that teeth and gums are isolated, mechanical parts of the body, and instead see the mouth as a living, responsive environment that reflects—and influences—our overall health. Rather than approaching oral care with a mindset of control and suppression, the natural philosophy invites partnership. It encourages us to work with the body's innate intelligence, support its balance, and foster conditions where healing can occur gently and sustainably over time.

This philosophy is grounded in respect: respect for the body's natural rhythms, for the microbial ecosystems that protect us, and for the traditional knowledge passed down through generations. Unlike the commercial dental model, which often promotes aggressive interventions and constant whitening, the natural approach is about creating health from within. It favors nourishment over punishment, observation over panic, and long-term well-being over short-term cosmetic fixes.

At the heart of this philosophy lies the principle that healing should be in harmony with nature. When we look at traditional practices from cultures around the world—Ayurvedic oil pulling, the use of herbal powders in African and Indigenous tribes, or the bamboo chewing sticks of the Middle East—we find a common theme: simplicity. These practices are not complicated, expensive, or high-tech, but they are effective because they respect the body's own healing mechanisms. They are rooted in daily rhythm, prevention, and care rather than crisis management.

Modern oral care products, while often useful in specific contexts, tend to focus on attacking bacteria and sterilizing the mouth. This might seem logical at first glance, but the oral microbiome, much like the gut microbiome, thrives on balance—not elimination. When we constantly disrupt this balance with antibacterial rinses, synthetic additives, or harsh abrasives, we may solve one problem temporarily but create others in the long term. A natural and sustainable philosophy takes into account not only what a product does in the short term, but how it affects the body's ecosystem as a whole.

One of the guiding ideas in this approach is the concept of terrain. In natural healing traditions, terrain refers to the internal environment of the body. A healthy terrain resists disease not because pathogens are absent, but because balance is strong. Applied to oral health, this means supporting strong enamel through mineral-rich nutrition, encouraging a balanced microbiome by avoiding unnecessary chemicals, and maintaining circulation through habits like gum massage and hydration. Instead of fighting the body, we create an environment in which healing becomes inevitable.

This philosophy also honors the importance of sustainability—not just environmentally, but personally. It's not sustainable to rely on expensive procedures or to feel constantly anxious about every dental symptom. Healing the mouth naturally means choosing methods that are realistic to maintain over time, using ingredients that are safe and accessible, and cultivating habits that become part of your lifestyle rather than a temporary fix. When oral care becomes a nourishing daily ritual instead of a chore or a reaction to fear, it builds resilience not just in the mouth but in the nervous system and mindset as well.

This approach does not reject modern dentistry or science. Instead, it seeks to integrate evidence-based insight with traditional wisdom, focusing on prevention, root causes, and the body's natural ability to regenerate when supported. It welcomes the role of professionals while also empowering the individual. Just as you can nourish your body with food, movement, and rest, you can care for your mouth with tools and routines that are gentle, effective, and deeply aligned with your values.

We'll continue by looking at the core elements that make this philosophy work in practice—from how you choose your products to how you think about the role of bacteria, inflammation, and healing over time. These ideas form the foundation for the rituals and routines that follow throughout this book.

This philosophy encourages slowing down and paying attention to signals from your body rather than rushing to silence symptoms. A bleeding gum line, for example, is not just an inconvenience but a message that inflammation is present and needs care. Sensitivity to cold or sweetness can reveal early mineral loss in enamel, allowing you to intervene before damage becomes severe. By approaching these signs with curiosity rather than fear, you learn to respond with supportive practices instead of harsh treatments that might provide short-term relief but disrupt balance in the long term.

A central theme of this approach is nourishment. The teeth and gums, like every other tissue in the body, rely on a steady supply of minerals, vitamins, and healthy fats to remain strong. Vitamin D influences calcium absorption, vitamin K2 directs that calcium to the right places, and magnesium supports the structural integrity of both bone and enamel. Rather than seeing oral care as something separate from diet, the natural philosophy invites you to connect what you eat with how your mouth feels. Whole foods rich in these nutrients—leafy greens, fermented foods, pastured dairy, nuts, and seeds—become tools for prevention and slow repair.

Equally important is how this philosophy relates to habits beyond food. Oral health is deeply affected by stress, sleep, and even breathing patterns. Mouth breathing during sleep dries the oral tissues and changes the microbiome, leading to bad breath and increased risk of decay. High stress levels raise cortisol, which can weaken immunity and delay healing. In this context, natural oral care is not simply about brushing with herbal toothpaste but about cultivating a lifestyle that supports the body's resilience as a whole. A few minutes of mindful breathing before bed, drinking enough water throughout the day, and prioritizing restorative sleep can have as much impact on gum health as any mouth rinse.

Sustainability also means understanding your relationship to consumer culture. Modern dental care often equates health with constant purchasing: specialized rinses for whitening, separate pastes for sensitivity, strips for quick cosmetic fixes. A natural philosophy encourages stepping back to question what is truly needed. Many effective solutions are simple, low-cost, and time-tested. A homemade rinse made from salt and warm water can soothe inflamed gums. A soft-bristled brush used consistently and with patience protects enamel better than aggressive whitening tools. By shifting focus from marketing-driven products to daily rhythms, you create a system that feels grounded and achievable.

This approach does not ask you to reject professional care. Dentists play a vital role in diagnosing, guiding, and treating issues that go beyond what at-home methods can address. Integrating natural care means using professional support wisely—choosing cleanings, checkups, and interventions when appropriate, while also understanding that the everyday choices you make between visits determine long-term outcomes. By building a foundation of natural habits, you arrive at appointments healthier and better informed, making treatments less frequent and less invasive.

The deeper reward of this philosophy is the relationship you develop with your own body. When you begin to care for your mouth naturally and sustainably, oral care stops feeling like a chore. It becomes an act of respect toward yourself, a way to connect with your body's signals and honor its needs. Over time, this practice can shift how you view health altogether. Instead of constantly reacting to problems, you start cultivating conditions for balance and vitality. The mouth, once treated as a separate system, becomes a trusted indicator of how well the whole body is being supported. In the chapters ahead, this perspective will guide each practical tool and routine. Whether exploring the role of the oral microbiome, experimenting with herbal rinses, or adjusting diet to support remineralization, every technique will reflect the same principle: gentle, informed care that works with your body rather than against it. This is what makes healing not only possible but sustainable for a lifetime.

How to Use This Book: Science Meets Tradition, Prevention Meets Healing

This book is designed to do more than teach you about oral health. Its purpose is to help you experience a shift in how you view your mouth and, ultimately, your entire body. Most people grow up thinking of oral care as a routine chore: brushing in the morning, flossing if they remember, and visiting the dentist twice a year. Rarely do we consider how deeply our mouths reflect our overall health or how time-tested traditions can enhance what modern research is only beginning to confirm. This book bridges those two worlds so you can draw from the strengths of both.

To make the most of what follows, it helps to understand the philosophy behind its structure. Each section moves in a deliberate sequence, starting with foundational insights and gradually layering practical applications. The early chapters explore why oral health matters far beyond the teeth and gums, establishing the profound connections between the mouth, the microbiome, and systemic wellbeing. Later chapters introduce specific tools and practices—dietary changes, herbal remedies, daily rituals—that integrate this knowledge into real life. By the time you finish, you will not only know what to do but also why it matters and how to adapt it to your own circumstances.

A Meeting of Two Worlds

The strength of this book lies in its union of tradition and science. Ancient practices such as oil pulling, gum massage, and herbal rinses have stood the test of time, practiced by cultures across continents for generations. These methods were born from observation and passed down because they worked. Modern research now offers a clearer lens, revealing how these same practices influence bacteria, inflammation, and even mineral balance in teeth. Understanding both perspectives allows you to practice oral care in a way that feels both grounded and informed.

This integration is important because relying exclusively on one side often leaves gaps. Traditional wisdom alone, while rich in experience, can sometimes lack the specificity needed to address unique modern challenges such as processed foods or environmental toxins. On the other hand, modern dentistry, while invaluable for acute care, can become overly focused on treating symptoms rather than supporting long-term balance. By combining the best of both, you are empowered to take preventive action while still knowing when professional help is needed.

Prevention and Healing as Partners

Most people think of prevention and healing as separate phases: you either maintain health or fix problems. In reality, the two constantly overlap. Preventive habits like mineral-rich nutrition and gentle daily care actively support healing, while the process of healing itself reveals what future prevention requires. This book treats them as partners. As you apply these practices, you may notice that what helps a sensitive tooth recover also protects it from future damage. The goal is to create routines that serve you in both states, so you no longer feel caught in cycles of neglect and crisis.

The chapters that follow are designed to guide you step by step. Some will explain concepts in depth, such as the oral microbiome and its role in whole-body health. Others will give practical tools, like how to prepare a simple herbal rinse or structure a daily oral care ritual that is realistic to maintain. Throughout, you will find explanations rooted in both tradition and current research, helping you understand the deeper reasons behind each recommendation.

As you move through the chapters, allow yourself to absorb the concepts gradually rather than rushing to implement everything at once. Some practices will resonate immediately and feel simple to adopt, while others may require reflection or small adjustments before they become part of your daily life. This is intentional. True healing happens in layers, and by pacing yourself, you give your body and mind the space to integrate change in a way that feels sustainable.

The structure of the book encourages flexibility. You can read it straight through to build a complete understanding of how natural oral healing works, or you can skip to the chapters that address your most pressing concerns, such as gum sensitivity, mineral loss, or balancing the microbiome. Each section is self-contained enough to stand alone, yet together they form a complete system that blends prevention and active healing. This means you can revisit the content multiple times, each reading offering new insights as your circumstances evolve.

Applying the material works best when you treat it as an ongoing dialogue with your own body. Notice how your gums respond to dietary changes, how your breath improves with daily tongue cleaning, or how sensitivity shifts when you begin using mineral-supportive remedies. These observations are not just feedback but guidance, showing you which habits are making the most difference and which may need refinement. Over time, this self-awareness helps you personalize the principles in this book to fit your lifestyle rather than forcing yourself into rigid routines.

One important aspect of this approach is respect for both modern dentistry and ancestral wisdom. You will learn how to integrate professional checkups and cleanings with natural care at home, understanding that each plays a role. Professional diagnostics can identify problems early, while the daily practices you adopt provide the foundation for long-term resilience. This synergy reduces the need for emergency interventions and helps you feel more confident in every choice you make about your oral health.

Throughout the book, references to research are included where they add clarity and reassurance. They are not meant to overwhelm with technical language but to validate practices that might otherwise seem unconventional. For example, when you read about oil pulling or the use of specific herbs, you will see how modern studies have explored their antimicrobial and anti-inflammatory properties, adding context to traditions that have been passed down for centuries. This balance allows you to trust both the wisdom of the past and the insights of current science without feeling pulled entirely toward one or the other.

The practical exercises, recipes, and routines offered are designed to be adaptable. If you have limited time, you can begin with a few core practices and expand later. If you are motivated to make bigger changes, you will find deeper guidance on building comprehensive routines and understanding the reasons behind them. What matters most is consistency rather than perfection. A single thoughtful practice performed daily will always create more lasting results than an overwhelming schedule you abandon after a week.

By approaching the book in this way, you create a foundation for change that feels empowering rather than burdensome. The following chapters invite you to explore the intimate connection between your mouth and your entire body, equipping you with knowledge and tools that honor both tradition and science. Each page is meant to guide you toward a healthier, more balanced relationship with your oral health—one that supports not just your teeth and gums but your overall vitality for years to come.

Part I. The Foundations of Oral Healing

Before diving into specific practices and routines, it is essential to understand the foundation on which natural oral healing rests. Without this base, even the best remedies or habits will feel scattered and disconnected. The goal of this first part is to help you see your mouth in a completely new way, shifting from isolated symptom management to a broader understanding of how oral health reflects and influences your entire body.

Most people are accustomed to viewing oral care as a simple checklist: brush, floss, visit the dentist twice a year. While these habits have value, they rarely address why problems arise in the first place or how daily choices ripple through the mouth and into systemic health. This part of the book aims to bridge that gap by exploring the deeper factors that shape oral wellness, including the relationship between the oral microbiome, inflammation, and lifestyle. It will give you the clarity needed to see oral health as part of whole-body care rather than a separate task.

These chapters begin by looking closely at the mouth as a gateway to overall vitality. You will discover how gum health connects to heart health, why the bacteria in your mouth can affect digestion and immunity, and how even subtle changes in oral balance can influence energy levels and mental clarity. The science here is compelling, but it is presented in a way that feels approachable, connecting research findings to practical realities you can see and feel in daily life.

At the same time, this section introduces you to ancestral perspectives on oral care. Many traditional practices—oil pulling, herbal rinses, tongue cleaning—emerged centuries ago from careful observation and lived experience. While modern dentistry often focuses on intervention, these older methods prioritized prevention and harmony with the body's natural rhythms. By exploring both, you will gain a balanced understanding that neither glorifies the past nor dismisses modern insights, but instead integrates them to create a more complete picture.

Another purpose of this part is to help you identify and unlearn common misconceptions. Much of what is marketed as oral care today prioritizes appearance over health or seeks quick fixes rather than addressing root causes. Through these chapters, you will see why over-sanitizing the mouth can backfire, why minerals matter more than whitening strips, and why sustainable habits always outperform extreme measures. This clarity will make it easier to discern which practices genuinely support your health and which simply create more dependency on products or procedures.

By the end of this section, you will have a new framework for thinking about oral health—one that respects the mouth as a vital part of your internal ecosystem and equips you to move forward with confidence. The knowledge you gain here will serve as the groundwork for everything that follows, ensuring that as you adopt specific remedies and rituals later in the book, they align with a deeper understanding of how healing truly happens. This is where your journey begins: with awareness, with respect for your body's intelligence, and with a commitment to building health that lasts.

Chapter 1: Why Your Mouth Is the Gateway to Your Health

The Oral–Systemic Connection: Gums, Inflammation, and Chronic Illness

The mouth is often treated as if it exists in isolation, separate from the rest of the body. Yet research and lived experience both reveal a different truth: the health of your gums and oral tissues is deeply intertwined with your overall wellbeing. The same blood that nourishes your heart, lungs, and brain flows through your mouth. The same immune system that defends you from infections elsewhere also responds to the bacterial balance in your gums. This interconnectedness explains why oral inflammation can influence chronic conditions and why addressing gum health can sometimes ease systemic strain.

The Biology of Connection

Gums are not just soft tissue framing the teeth; they are active participants in your immune and circulatory systems. When gum tissue becomes inflamed—a condition known as gingivitis in its early stages and periodontitis when more advanced—it triggers a cascade of immune responses. Inflammation increases blood flow to the affected area to deliver white blood cells and nutrients, which is the body's attempt to heal. However, when this state of heightened immune activity becomes chronic, it stops being protective and begins to harm.

Harmful bacteria that thrive in inflamed gums can release toxins into the bloodstream. Small tears in gum tissue, which often occur during brushing or flossing in individuals with gum disease, provide direct pathways for these microbes and inflammatory molecules to travel beyond the mouth. Studies, including those reviewed by Di Stefano (2022), highlight how specific pathogens like *Porphyromonas gingivalis* have been found not only in oral infections but also in distant tissues, including arterial plaques. This suggests that gum disease may contribute to the progression of cardiovascular conditions by fueling low-grade systemic inflammation.

Inflammation as a Common Thread

Chronic inflammation is now recognized as a key factor in many modern illnesses: heart disease, diabetes, autoimmune disorders, and even certain neurological conditions. Oral inflammation feeds into this broader picture. Elevated levels of C-reactive protein (CRP), an inflammatory marker, are commonly observed in both periodontal disease and cardiovascular disease, pointing to shared biological pathways. While gum disease does not single-handedly cause heart attacks or strokes, it adds to the total inflammatory burden, making it harder for the body to maintain balance.

Diabetes provides another example of this two-way relationship. High blood sugar levels weaken the immune response and make gum tissue more susceptible to infection. In turn, oral inflammation can worsen insulin resistance, creating a feedback loop where both conditions aggravate each other. This is why comprehensive diabetes management increasingly includes regular periodontal assessments and why improving gum health can support better blood sugar control.

A Broader Impact Than We Realize

The connection between oral health and chronic illness is not limited to the heart and metabolism. Research continues to explore links to respiratory conditions, adverse pregnancy outcomes, and even cognitive decline. Harmful oral bacteria have been detected in the lungs of individuals with chronic obstructive pulmonary disease, suggesting aspiration of bacteria from the mouth may play a role. Pregnant individuals with untreated gum disease are at higher risk for preterm birth and low birth weight, likely due to systemic inflammatory signals reaching the placenta.

These findings are significant because they shift how we think about oral care. Instead of viewing gum health as separate from overall health, we can start seeing it as part of a whole-body strategy for prevention and healing. Strengthening gum integrity, balancing oral bacteria, and reducing chronic inflammation may support far more than a healthy smile; it may influence energy levels, immune resilience, and long-term vitality.

Understanding this relationship between the gums and systemic health makes it clear why even small improvements in daily care can have profound ripple effects. Reducing chronic inflammation in the mouth lightens the workload of the immune system, freeing up resources for healing and maintaining balance elsewhere in the body. This is why some people notice broader benefits—better energy, improved digestion, or fewer flare-ups of inflammatory conditions—once they begin paying consistent attention to oral care beyond the basics of brushing and flossing.

The first step is recognizing inflammation early rather than waiting for severe symptoms to appear. Gums that bleed during brushing, persistent bad breath, or a slight swelling around the gumline are often dismissed as minor issues. In reality, they are early warning signs of imbalance. Addressing them promptly with gentle but consistent practices can prevent progression and reduce the likelihood of systemic impact. This is not about panic or self-diagnosis but about developing an awareness of how the mouth signals what is happening inside the body.

Practical changes to calm gum inflammation begin with creating a stable environment for the oral microbiome. Choosing a toothpaste that avoids harsh antibacterials, incorporating mineral-rich foods like leafy greens and fermented dairy, and maintaining proper hydration can all contribute to a healthier oral terrain. Natural approaches such as herbal rinses with ingredients like neem or clove can support balance without over-sanitizing, while oil pulling has been shown in studies like Kaushik et al. (2016) to reduce harmful bacteria such as *Streptococcus mutans*. These gentle practices work by supporting the body's natural defenses rather than attempting to sterilize the mouth entirely, which can often backfire by disrupting beneficial flora.

Equally important is how lifestyle factors outside the mouth affect gum health. Chronic stress is a major driver of inflammation, weakening immune function and slowing healing in oral tissues. Prioritizing restorative sleep, incorporating stress-reducing practices like deep breathing or walking outdoors, and ensuring steady blood sugar levels through balanced meals can all influence gum resilience. For individuals managing conditions like diabetes, integrating oral care into the broader framework of metabolic health often leads to better outcomes in both areas.

Professional care also remains a vital part of this equation. Natural healing does not mean avoiding dentists but working in partnership with them. Regular checkups can catch issues that daily observation might miss, and professional cleanings remove hardened plaque that cannot be addressed at home. Combining these visits with informed daily routines creates a synergy: the dentist addresses what you cannot, while your habits maintain balance between appointments. This cooperative approach respects the strengths of both modern dentistry and natural methods, ensuring you benefit from the best of each.

The bigger shift comes in mindset. When you begin viewing your gums as part of a larger system rather than an isolated concern, oral care transforms from a task to a form of whole-body prevention. Each choice—what you eat, how you manage stress, how you nurture microbial balance—becomes an investment in long-term vitality rather than a reaction to immediate problems. This perspective reduces anxiety around oral health because it equips you with tools and understanding rather than leaving you dependent on emergency fixes.

By the end of this book, you will have a clear framework for applying this knowledge in daily life. The chapters ahead will guide you through specific practices, from dietary strategies that strengthen gum tissue to rituals like tongue cleaning and gum massage that improve circulation and microbial balance. These are not quick fixes but sustainable habits that evolve with you. In learning to care for your mouth naturally and consistently, you will also be caring for your heart, your immune system, and your overall wellbeing in ways you may not have realized were possible.

The Forgotten Microbiome: Balancing "Good" and "Bad" Bacteria in the Mouth

Few people realize that their mouths host one of the most diverse microbial ecosystems in the human body. More than 700 species of bacteria, along with fungi and other microorganisms, live on the tongue, gums, teeth, and even within saliva. For decades, dental care was primarily focused on eradicating bacteria, assuming that a sterile mouth was a healthy mouth. Yet modern research paints a different picture: the goal is not to eliminate bacteria but to maintain balance between helpful and harmful species. When harmony is preserved, these microorganisms contribute to strong teeth, healthy gums, and even digestive and immune health. When balance is lost, oral disease and systemic inflammation can follow.

The concept of an oral microbiome is similar to the better-known gut microbiome, which has received significant attention in recent years for its role in immunity and mental health. Like the gut, the oral microbiome thrives on diversity and cooperation. Beneficial bacteria help neutralize acids, support remineralization of teeth, and compete with harmful organisms for space and resources. Disrupting this community through harsh antibacterial rinses, constant sugar exposure, or processed foods can tip the scales, allowing opportunistic species to dominate and cause damage.

Why Balance Matters

The bacteria considered "bad" are not inherently malicious; many live peacefully in small numbers without causing harm. Problems arise when conditions favor their overgrowth. For instance, *Streptococcus mutans* thrives in high-sugar environments, producing acid that erodes enamel and leads to cavities. Similarly, anaerobic bacteria like *Porphyromonas gingivalis* can trigger gum inflammation when oral hygiene or immune defenses falter. On the other hand, beneficial bacteria such as *Streptococcus salivarius* can produce compounds that inhibit pathogens and help maintain a neutral pH. The dynamic between these organisms is constantly shifting in response to diet, stress, hydration, and overall health.

Understanding this balance changes how we approach oral care. Rather than aiming to sterilize the mouth, the focus shifts to creating conditions where beneficial bacteria thrive and harmful ones remain in check. This means supporting the ecosystem rather than waging war against it. It also means recognizing that the mouth is not separate from the rest of the body: a disrupted oral microbiome can affect digestion, immunity, and even the gut, since bacteria from the mouth are swallowed daily.

The Role of Diet and Lifestyle

What you eat profoundly influences the oral microbiome. Diets high in refined sugars and processed carbohydrates fuel acid-producing bacteria, while mineral-rich foods and fibrous vegetables encourage salivary flow and promote balance. Micronutrients like vitamin D, calcium, and vitamin K2 play critical roles in strengthening enamel and supporting healthy bone around the teeth, indirectly shaping the microbial environment by making it less hospitable to harmful species. Hydration matters as well; saliva not only washes away food particles but also carries enzymes and antimicrobial peptides that keep the ecosystem in equilibrium.

Lifestyle habits extend beyond food. Stress, for instance, can alter the immune system and reduce saliva production, creating an environment where harmful bacteria multiply more easily. Poor sleep has similar effects, and mouth breathing can further dry oral tissues, shifting the microbial landscape toward imbalance. Even oral hygiene practices themselves play a role: overly aggressive brushing or the frequent use of strong antibacterial mouthwashes may disrupt beneficial bacteria and create a rebound effect where harmful organisms repopulate faster.

Practical ways to support this microbial balance begin with restoring a healthy environment rather than targeting individual species. Saliva is one of the body's most powerful tools for this purpose. It buffers acids, delivers minerals like calcium and phosphate for remineralization, and contains natural antimicrobial compounds that keep populations of harmful bacteria under control. Staying hydrated, chewing fibrous foods, and even mindful chewing itself can stimulate saliva flow, providing constant support to the oral ecosystem.

Herbal remedies can also play a role when chosen thoughtfully. Neem, clove, and myrrh have long histories in traditional oral care and modern studies confirm their antibacterial and anti-inflammatory properties. When used in gentle rinses or tooth powders, they help control harmful bacteria without wiping out beneficial strains. This selective action is crucial: unlike synthetic antiseptics that attempt to sterilize, plant-based compounds often work in harmony with the microbiome, nudging it back toward balance rather than forcing a total reset.

Oil pulling offers another example of this principle in action. Research such as the randomized controlled trial by Kaushik et al. (2016) found that daily swishing with coconut oil reduced *Streptococcus mutans* levels in saliva to a degree comparable to chlorhexidine rinses. Unlike strong chemical mouthwashes, oil pulling does not disrupt the entire microbial community, and it adds the benefit of lubricating oral tissues and gently massaging the gums. It is not a cure-all, but it is a valuable adjunctive practice that supports the larger aim of balance.

Dietary strategies further reinforce microbial harmony. Including probiotic-rich foods like yogurt, kefir, or fermented vegetables can introduce beneficial bacteria that may influence oral and gut health alike. Prebiotic foods, particularly those rich in fiber, provide fuel for these helpful microbes. Limiting frequent snacking on refined carbohydrates reduces the constant acid challenge that fuels decay-causing bacteria, allowing saliva to restore pH and protect enamel between meals.

Beyond food and remedies, awareness of early signs of imbalance is equally important. Persistent bad breath, metallic taste, or recurring gum tenderness can indicate a shift toward harmful bacterial dominance. Rather than masking these symptoms, viewing them as feedback encourages gentle course correction. Adding an extra session of tongue cleaning, increasing hydration, or adjusting dietary choices can often restore balance before problems escalate.

Integrating these practices does not require perfection or drastic lifestyle changes. Small, consistent actions create an environment where beneficial bacteria naturally thrive. Choosing toothpaste without harsh antibacterials, rinsing with salt water after meals, and prioritizing whole foods over processed snacks are simple shifts that build momentum over time. As these habits settle into routine, their impact extends beyond oral health. A balanced microbiome reduces chronic inflammation, supports immune function, and even influences digestion since every swallow carries oral bacteria into the gut.

The broader reward of caring for this forgotten ecosystem is the relationship it fosters with your own body. Instead of seeing bacteria as enemies, you begin to understand them as partners that respond to how you live and what you provide for them. This shift transforms oral care from a reactive chore into an act of stewardship, one that not only protects your teeth and gums but also nurtures the interconnected systems that sustain overall health.

How Modern Habits Silently Damage Oral Health (Diet, Stress, Chemicals)

Most people assume oral problems begin with obvious triggers, like forgetting to brush or indulging in too many sweets. In reality, the decline in oral health often starts quietly, shaped by everyday habits that seem harmless but slowly shift the balance of the mouth's ecosystem. Diet, stress, and chemical exposure all influence how bacteria behave, how enamel repairs itself, and how gums respond to irritation. Over time, these factors create conditions where cavities, gum disease, and chronic inflammation can take root without dramatic warning signs. Understanding these subtle influences is essential if you want to stop problems before they begin.

Diet: More Than Just Sugar

Sugar's link to tooth decay is well known, but modern diets present more complex challenges than a simple candy habit. Highly processed foods dominate most grocery shelves and contain refined starches that quickly break down into sugars in the mouth. These sticky residues feed acid-producing bacteria, lowering oral pH and initiating enamel demineralization. Unlike whole foods, which are chewed thoroughly and stimulate saliva production, processed snacks often require little chewing and leave a film that clings to teeth and gums. This lingering acidity erodes enamel gradually, often without pain until significant damage has occurred.

Equally significant is the lack of protective nutrients in modern diets. Vitamins A, D, and K2, along with minerals like calcium and magnesium, are critical for remineralizing enamel and maintaining healthy gum tissue. When these nutrients are insufficient, the body struggles to repair daily microscopic damage. Traditional diets rich in organ meats, fermented foods, and mineral-dense vegetables naturally supported oral resilience. Today, even individuals who avoid obvious junk food can miss these key nutrients, leaving their teeth more vulnerable to wear and decay.

Frequent snacking further compounds the issue. Every time food is consumed, bacteria metabolize sugars and release acids. If eating happens every hour, the mouth never returns to a neutral pH, and enamel remains under near-constant attack. This pattern, common with modern grazing habits and sugary beverages, silently undermines tooth strength despite seemingly adequate brushing and flossing.

Stress: The Invisible Saboteur

Modern life is marked by chronic stress, and its effects on oral health are often underestimated. Stress triggers cortisol release, which can suppress immune function and slow tissue repair. This makes gums more susceptible to inflammation and less able to heal after minor irritation. Over time, this low-level stress response contributes to gingivitis and, in more severe cases, periodontitis.

Stress also changes behavior in ways that harm oral health. Jaw clenching and teeth grinding, often occurring during sleep, can wear down enamel and create microfractures. These habits may not be noticed until sensitivity or visible cracks appear. Additionally, stress can dry the mouth by reducing saliva flow, allowing harmful bacteria to multiply unchecked. A dry mouth not only feels uncomfortable but also accelerates cavity formation and bad breath.

The connection between emotional state and oral health is cyclical. Gum problems or visible damage to teeth can create anxiety about appearance or health, which in turn fuels more stress. Breaking this cycle requires recognizing the influence of psychological factors on physical wellbeing and addressing both rather than focusing solely on mechanical cleaning.

Chemical exposure is another factor that quietly reshapes the oral environment, often in ways that are misunderstood. Many conventional oral care products, while marketed as protective, rely on strong antibacterial agents or synthetic additives that can disrupt the very balance they are meant to maintain. Ingredients like triclosan, once common in toothpaste and mouthwash, have been shown to reduce bacterial diversity and potentially contribute to resistance in microbes. Sodium lauryl sulfate, a foaming agent, can irritate soft tissues and worsen conditions like canker sores. Even constant use of alcohol-based mouthwashes may dry the oral tissues, removing the natural lubrication that saliva provides and creating an environment where harmful bacteria can repopulate quickly.

Fluoride is another widely discussed element in modern oral care. While fluoride can strengthen enamel and has a well-documented role in reducing cavities, concerns arise from its overuse. Excessive exposure, particularly in children, can contribute to dental fluorosis, a condition marked by changes in tooth enamel appearance. The key is not complete avoidance but mindful use, understanding that more is not always better and that the context of diet and mineral intake matters. Balanced fluoride exposure, combined with nutrient-rich foods that naturally support remineralization, often offers better results than relying solely on fortified products.

Beyond oral care products, environmental chemicals also influence gum and tooth health. Pesticide residues, plasticizers like BPA found in certain food packaging, and heavy metals from water sources can accumulate in the body and subtly affect immune function and inflammatory responses. These exposures do not cause immediate pain or visible damage, which is why they often go unnoticed. Over time, however, they may contribute to chronic inflammation that weakens gum integrity and alters microbial balance. Reducing these exposures through filtered water, glass or stainless-steel storage, and choosing whole, minimally processed foods supports not only oral health but general wellbeing.

Recognizing these influences allows for a more nuanced approach to care. Instead of focusing only on cleaning teeth or removing bacteria, the priority becomes creating conditions where balance is restored and maintained. This means choosing oral care products with gentle, non-disruptive ingredients, paying attention to hydration and mineral intake, and managing stress in ways that calm the body's inflammatory responses. It also involves understanding that health is cumulative: small daily decisions, whether about food, sleep, or the products we use, gradually shape the mouth's ability to stay resilient.

Practical steps can begin with awareness. Reading ingredient labels, spacing meals to allow natural pH recovery, and incorporating relaxation techniques into daily routines may seem simple, yet their combined effect is profound. These actions do not merely address surface-level problems like plaque or bad breath but help transform the internal environment so issues are less likely to arise in the first place. The shift is subtle at first—a decrease in gum tenderness, fresher breath upon waking—but over months it builds into long-term stability.

Embracing this perspective is empowering. It reframes oral care as something you actively shape rather than something done to you during biannual dental visits. By addressing diet, stress, and chemical exposures together, you move beyond isolated fixes toward a lifestyle that naturally supports the body's own healing mechanisms. This integrated approach does more than protect teeth and gums; it contributes to systemic balance, making oral wellness a meaningful part of overall health rather than an afterthought.

Chapter 2: Ancient Wisdom vs. Modern Dentistry

Traditional Practices Across Cultures (Ayurveda, Chinese, Indigenous)

Throughout human history, cultures across the world have developed their own methods of caring for the mouth, long before modern dentistry existed. These practices emerged from observation, experience, and a deep understanding of the relationship between oral health and overall vitality. While their language and concepts differed, a unifying thread connects them: the belief that the mouth reflects the state of the whole body and that tending to it supports balance far beyond the teeth and gums.

Ayurvedic Traditions

Ayurveda, the ancient healing system of India, has one of the most detailed approaches to oral care found in traditional medicine. Central to this system is the idea that oral health is inseparable from systemic balance, or dosha harmony. Daily routines, known as *dinacharya*, include practices specifically designed to cleanse and nourish the mouth.

One of the most recognizable Ayurvedic practices is oil pulling, referred to as *kavala* or *gandusha*. This involves swishing sesame or coconut oil in the mouth for several minutes each morning to draw out impurities, lubricate tissues, and support the oral microbiome. Modern studies have found that oil pulling can reduce harmful bacteria such as *Streptococcus mutans* and help decrease plaque buildup, confirming some of what practitioners observed centuries ago.

Ayurveda also recommends tongue scraping with a copper or stainless-steel scraper. This removes accumulated coatings, or *ama*, believed to represent toxins from digestion. From a modern perspective, tongue scraping reduces bacterial load on the tongue's surface and improves breath freshness. Herbal powders made from neem, clove, and licorice were also used to massage the gums and clean the teeth, offering antimicrobial and anti-inflammatory benefits.

Chinese Medicine and Oral Care

Traditional Chinese Medicine (TCM) also views the mouth as a reflection of internal health. In this system, each tooth is connected through meridians to specific organs, suggesting that imbalances in the liver, kidneys, or heart may reveal themselves through changes in oral tissues. While these correspondences are not literal in modern scientific terms, the holistic observation behind them often pointed practitioners toward systemic causes of oral problems, such as digestive weakness or chronic inflammation.

Oral hygiene practices in ancient China included the use of herbal rinses and chewing sticks. Green tea, known for its antioxidant and antibacterial properties, was used both as a beverage and a mouth rinse to freshen breath and reduce plaque. Licorice root and honeysuckle were applied for soothing inflamed gums. In some regions, salt water rinses were common, a practice still recommended today for their ability to cleanse gently and support healing without disrupting the oral microbiome.

Chinese dietary therapy also addressed oral health indirectly. Foods rich in minerals and cooling properties were believed to support gum integrity and reduce inflammation. Excessive consumption of sugar, though rare in traditional diets, was discouraged as it was thought to generate "damp heat," a state linked to decay and infection.

Among Indigenous cultures, oral care was inseparable from the land and the resources it provided. Communities in North America, Africa, and Australia each developed distinct methods rooted in the plants, clays, and fibers available to them. Chewing sticks were among the most widespread tools. These were typically cut from twigs with natural antibacterial properties, such as miswak from the Salvadora persica tree in parts of Africa and the Middle East. The fibers of the twig would fray as it was chewed, forming a brush-like texture that could clean teeth and massage gums without damaging enamel. Studies conducted in modern times have confirmed the antimicrobial effects of miswak, validating the effectiveness of a tool in use for centuries.

Other Indigenous traditions relied on ashes, charcoals, or finely ground clays to clean teeth and neutralize acids in the mouth. In some cultures, burnt herbs or wood were combined with animal fats or plant oils to form rudimentary pastes that doubled as both cleaners and breath fresheners.

While these mixtures lacked the convenience of modern toothpaste, they provided mild abrasiveness to remove plaque and incorporated minerals that supported enamel strength.

The use of plants for healing inflamed or infected gums was also common. In many North American tribes, for instance, willow bark was chewed not only for its cleansing effect but also for its natural salicin content, which provided mild pain relief and reduced inflammation. Similarly, certain roots and barks with bitter or astringent qualities were used to tighten gum tissue and promote healing. These remedies were discovered through close observation of nature and refined over generations, often becoming part of daily life rather than reserved for times of illness.

A striking feature of Indigenous oral care is the absence of separation between food, medicine, and hygiene. Nutrient-dense diets rich in unprocessed animal and plant foods naturally supported oral health, providing vitamins A, D, and K2, as well as minerals like calcium and phosphorus. Fermented foods and seasonal diversity helped maintain microbial balance, while the lack of refined sugar protected against the bacterial overgrowth that drives cavities and gum disease. The very act of eating tougher, fibrous foods contributed to mechanical cleaning of teeth and stimulated saliva flow, reducing the need for elaborate oral care routines.

These practices illustrate a principle that runs through many traditional systems: oral health was maintained by living in alignment with the environment rather than relying on isolated interventions. Cleaning methods were simple but effective, and dietary patterns worked in harmony with natural rhythms. Modern lifestyles often lack this synergy, which is why revisiting these ancestral insights can feel like uncovering forgotten truths rather than adopting something foreign or extreme.

Integrating these approaches into contemporary life does not require abandoning modern dentistry. Instead, it invites us to borrow what is still relevant: gentle cleaning methods that respect the microbiome, the use of herbal rinses or oils to soothe and balance, and the prioritization of nutrient-rich foods as the foundation of oral health. When paired with professional care and current research, these practices create a more complete model of wellness—one that honors both tradition and innovation.

How Industrial Marketing Replaced Generations of Natural Wisdom

For most of human history, oral care relied on simple practices rooted in observation and local resources. People cleaned their teeth with twigs, rinsed with salt water or herbal infusions, and ate diets naturally supportive of gum and tooth health. These habits were not perfect, but they worked in harmony with the body and rarely conflicted with the oral microbiome. The shift away from this wisdom began gradually during the industrial era, accelerating in the twentieth century when mass marketing transformed not only how people cleaned their teeth but how they thought about oral health altogether.

The Rise of Commercial Oral Care

The industrial revolution made it possible to mass-produce toothpaste, toothbrushes, and mouthwashes. Initially, this was a practical advancement: products became more affordable and widely available. But as companies competed for market share, marketing strategies began to focus less on health and more on creating consumer desire. Advertisements linked fresh breath and bright white teeth to attractiveness, success, and social acceptance. Oral care was reframed from a holistic health practice to a cosmetic ritual, shifting the priority from supporting natural balance to achieving a polished appearance.

This change was subtle but profound. For centuries, oral health had been inseparable from diet and lifestyle. Nutrient-dense foods, natural cleaning methods, and seasonal rhythms maintained balance without heavy intervention. With industrial marketing, attention shifted toward products that promised quick fixes—whitening pastes, antiseptic rinses, and flavored powders—while the role of nutrition and gentle care faded from public consciousness. The idea that the body could heal and maintain itself was overshadowed by the message that external products were essential for cleanliness and confidence.

The Whitening Obsession

One of the clearest examples of this shift is the emphasis on whiteness as a marker of health. Historically, tooth color varied naturally and mild staining was common, especially in cultures consuming mineral-rich foods and herbal preparations. Industrial marketing, however, equated bright white teeth with vitality and moral virtue. Companies launched aggressive campaigns suggesting that anything less was unattractive or unclean.

This narrative drove the development of abrasives and bleaching agents in toothpaste, some of which were harsh enough to wear down enamel over time. While these products created the illusion of health by polishing surface stains, they often ignored deeper issues such as gum health or mineral balance. As consumers sought ever-whiter smiles, they became more reliant on commercial solutions, perpetuating a cycle of cosmetic concern rather than true healing.

Antibacterial Extremes

Another turning point came with the marketing of antiseptic mouthwashes. In the early twentieth century, companies promoted alcohol-based rinses as essential for killing "germs" and preventing bad breath. While these products did reduce odor temporarily, they also disrupted the delicate ecosystem of the mouth. Beneficial bacteria were swept away alongside harmful ones, often leaving the environment more vulnerable to imbalance once recolonization occurred.

The focus on sterilization ignored a key principle of oral health: balance rather than eradication. Traditional methods like oil pulling or herbal rinses aimed to support harmony in the mouth, not destroy it. Industrial marketing reframed bacteria as enemies to be eliminated at all costs, a message that still dominates advertising today. This oversimplification fueled decades of practices that stripped the mouth of its natural defenses in the name of cleanliness.

The impact of this marketing shift extended beyond products to the way people understood the causes of oral disease. As companies promoted toothpaste and mouthwash as the primary solutions, the role of diet and lifestyle was downplayed or forgotten altogether. Generations grew up believing cavities were the result of poor brushing habits rather than deficiencies in minerals, chronic inflammation, or the effects of processed foods. This misunderstanding allowed the food industry to expand its use of refined sugars and additives with little scrutiny, while the dental industry provided treatments and products to manage the consequences rather than address the root causes.

Nutritional pioneers of the early twentieth century, such as Weston A. Price, documented how indigenous communities with traditional diets enjoyed remarkably low rates of tooth decay and gum disease. Their oral health deteriorated rapidly only after adopting processed flour, sugar, and canned foods. Yet these observations rarely influenced mainstream dental care because they conflicted with the commercial narrative that products, rather than whole foods and lifestyle, were the key to oral health. The result was a widening gap between what ancestral knowledge suggested and what consumers were taught through advertising.

Over time, this gap fostered dependency. Instead of trusting their bodies to maintain balance through proper nourishment and gentle daily care, people came to view oral health as something that required constant intervention by products. Whitening strips, antibacterial rinses, and specialty toothpastes promised solutions to problems they often helped create in the first place. The message was consistent: more is better, stronger is better, and without these products, your mouth is vulnerable. This mindset not only overlooked the body's natural capacity for healing but also encouraged overuse of substances that can disrupt the very systems they claim to protect.

The cultural consequences of this shift are subtle but significant. Oral care became less about prevention and more about appearance. The natural color and texture of teeth were pathologized, and mild staining from nutrient-rich foods or herbal remedies was framed as something shameful. At the same time, the deeper indicators of health—gum integrity, absence of chronic inflammation, balanced microbiota—received little attention in popular messaging. By redefining health as cosmetic perfection, industrial marketing diverted focus away from the practices that truly sustain oral and systemic wellness.

Reclaiming older wisdom does not mean rejecting every modern advancement. Fluoride, professional cleanings, and certain restorative treatments have undeniably improved outcomes in many cases. The key is discernment: understanding when modern interventions are appropriate and when ancestral principles offer safer, equally effective alternatives. For instance, incorporating mineral-rich foods, using gentle herbal rinses, and maintaining balance in the oral microbiome can complement professional care, reducing reliance on aggressive chemicals and constant whitening.

Bringing this awareness back into daily life begins with questioning assumptions. Why do we believe that every bacterium must be killed? Why do we equate whiter teeth with healthier teeth? And why do we rarely hear about the role of nutrition in preventing oral disease? Asking these questions opens the door to a more holistic approach—one that integrates the best of traditional and modern knowledge while respecting the body's innate wisdom. When oral care is reframed in this way, it stops being a cycle of endless products and becomes part of a broader commitment to whole-body health and sustainable living.

Lessons Modern Science Is Now Confirming from Ancient Oral Care

For centuries, traditional oral care practices were passed down through observation and experience. These methods—oil pulling, chewing sticks, herbal powders, tongue scraping—were rooted in daily routines and a deep understanding of nature. Long before modern dentistry, people noticed that these practices supported strong teeth, fresh breath, and overall vitality. Today, scientific research is beginning to validate what many ancient cultures already understood: the mouth is an ecosystem that thrives on balance, and simple, nature-based habits can have profound effects on oral health.

Oil Pulling and Its Validated Benefits

Oil pulling, most famously practiced in Ayurveda, is one of the clearest examples of ancient wisdom gaining modern recognition. The technique involves swishing oil—traditionally sesame, though coconut is now widely used—in the mouth for several minutes. Practitioners believed this helped "draw out toxins," lubricate tissues, and maintain oral cleanliness.

Modern studies, though framed in different language, confirm several of these benefits. Research by Kaushik et al. (2016) demonstrated that daily coconut oil pulling significantly reduced *Streptococcus mutans*, a primary bacteria responsible for tooth decay, with results comparable to chlorhexidine mouthwash. Additional studies have found reductions in plaque scores and improvements in gum health, likely due to the oil's antimicrobial and anti-inflammatory properties. While oil pulling is not a replacement for brushing and flossing, it serves as a gentle adjunctive practice that supports a healthy microbiome rather than disrupting it.

Herbal Antimicrobials: Neem, Clove, and Myrrh

Many cultures incorporated herbs into their oral care routines, not simply for flavor but for their medicinal properties. Neem, used extensively in India, was chewed as a twig or ground into powder for brushing. Clove and myrrh, valued for their analgesic and antiseptic qualities, were applied directly to soothe toothaches and inflamed gums.

Modern analysis reveals why these plants were so effective. Neem contains compounds with antibacterial and antifungal properties that inhibit cavity-causing and gum disease–related pathogens. Clove oil's eugenol content provides both pain relief and antimicrobial action, while myrrh has demonstrated wound-healing properties that support gum tissue repair. Studies like Bansal et al. (2020) show that these herbal extracts can inhibit *S. mutans* and *Candida albicans* growth in laboratory settings, lending scientific support to practices that persisted for generations.

Tongue Cleaning and Oral–Systemic Health

Tongue scraping, another cornerstone of Ayurvedic and East Asian oral care, was traditionally believed to remove toxins and improve digestion. Today, science offers a complementary explanation: the tongue harbors a significant portion of the mouth's bacterial load, and regular cleaning reduces compounds that contribute to bad breath and may influence oral pH.

Emerging research suggests that reducing tongue biofilm can also lower the bacterial load entering the digestive tract and potentially decrease the risk of systemic inflammation. While more studies are needed, the convergence between traditional reasoning and modern findings is striking. What was once viewed as a ritual of cleanliness is now recognized as a legitimate tool for microbiome support and preventive care.

Dietary patterns from ancestral cultures also reveal lessons that modern science continues to affirm. Traditional diets were naturally rich in fat-soluble vitamins such as A, D, and K2, along with minerals like calcium, phosphorus, and magnesium. These nutrients are essential for maintaining strong enamel and supporting the ongoing process of remineralization that occurs in the mouth. Weston A. Price's research in the early 20th century documented how isolated communities consuming unprocessed foods—wild fish, pasture-raised meats, fermented dairy, and seasonal vegetables—displayed wide dental arches, minimal crowding, and extremely low rates of cavities. When these populations transitioned to refined flours and sugars, dental decay and gum disease appeared within a single generation. Modern studies confirm this observation, linking nutrient density and low sugar intake to better oral and systemic health outcomes.

Mechanical cleaning methods used historically also offer valuable insight. Chewing sticks like miswak, derived from the Salvadora persica tree, were widely used in Africa, the Middle East, and parts of Asia. They served both as a toothbrush and a natural antibacterial tool, thanks to compounds like fluoride, silica, and sulfur present in the plant fibers. Studies comparing miswak users to conventional toothbrush users have found similar or even superior plaque control and gum health among those using the traditional method when applied correctly. Beyond their cleaning ability, these tools also stimulated saliva and gently massaged the gums, benefits that are often overlooked in modern oral care.

The simplicity of these ancestral routines is a key lesson. Instead of focusing on sterilizing the mouth or achieving unnaturally white teeth, traditional practices emphasized balance and maintenance. Cleaning was gentle yet consistent, nourishment came from whole foods rather than supplements, and oral health was seen as inseparable from overall vitality. Modern science is now catching up to this holistic view, with growing research on the oral microbiome, the impact of diet on enamel health, and the role of chronic inflammation in systemic disease.

Integrating these findings does not mean abandoning modern tools like toothbrushes or professional care. Rather, it suggests that combining ancestral practices with evidence-based dentistry can create a more complete approach. A daily routine might include brushing with a gentle, mineral-rich paste, using a tongue scraper, occasionally practicing oil pulling, and prioritizing nutrient-dense meals. These steps do not require expensive products or complicated regimens but instead encourage alignment with the body's natural rhythms and healing mechanisms.

The value of these lessons lies not only in their practicality but also in their ability to shift perspective. By understanding how older methods support what science now confirms, you begin to see oral care as less about quick fixes and more about long-term balance. This change in mindset reduces reliance on aggressive treatments and fosters respect for the body's inherent wisdom. When combined thoughtfully with modern knowledge, these practices provide a foundation for oral health that is sustainable, ethical, and deeply connected to overall wellbeing.

Chapter 3: The Hidden Toxins in Everyday Oral Care

Fluoride, Triclosan, SLS: What the Research Really Says

Modern oral care products often rely on a few key chemical ingredients that dominate mainstream toothpaste and mouthwash formulas: fluoride, triclosan, and sodium lauryl sulfate (SLS). These compounds have been widely used for decades, promoted as essential for cavity prevention, antibacterial protection, and foaming action. Yet their long-term effects and safety profiles continue to be debated, with research offering both support and caution. Understanding what science actually says about these ingredients allows for informed choices that align with both effectiveness and overall wellbeing.

Fluoride: Effective but Context Matters

Fluoride is arguably the most studied ingredient in oral care. Its primary benefit lies in strengthening enamel and reducing cavity risk by enhancing remineralization and making teeth more resistant to acid attacks. Community water fluoridation, introduced in the mid-20th century, contributed to a significant decline in tooth decay rates in many countries. Numerous studies, including large-scale reviews by organizations like the Cochrane Collaboration, confirm that fluoride can reduce cavity incidence by 20 to 40 percent when used appropriately.

However, the conversation is more nuanced than simply labeling fluoride as good or bad. While beneficial in controlled doses, overexposure can lead to dental fluorosis, a cosmetic condition where enamel develops white or brown streaks due to excessive fluoride during tooth development. Severe cases are rare, but mild fluorosis is relatively common in areas with naturally high fluoride in water or when multiple fluoride sources are combined, such as toothpaste, supplements, and mouth rinses.

There is also ongoing discussion about systemic versus topical fluoride. Many experts now suggest that the protective effects come primarily from direct contact with the teeth rather than ingestion. This raises questions about the necessity of water fluoridation in areas where topical products are widely used. For individuals aiming to minimize systemic exposure, using a fluoride toothpaste while avoiding unnecessary supplements or high-fluoride water may strike a balance between cavity protection and cautious use.

Triclosan: From Antibacterial Hero to Regulatory Scrutiny

Triclosan, once hailed for its potent antibacterial properties, was commonly added to toothpaste and mouthwash to reduce plaque and gingivitis. Early research supported its ability to lower gum inflammation and bacterial load. However, concerns emerged over its broader impact on health and the environment. Studies suggested that triclosan could disrupt hormone regulation in animals, contribute to antibiotic resistance, and persist in waterways, affecting aquatic ecosystems.

These findings prompted regulatory action. In 2016, the U.S. Food and Drug Administration banned triclosan in over-the-counter antibacterial soaps, citing insufficient evidence of additional benefits compared to regular soap and water and potential long-term risks. While this ban did not extend to toothpaste, several major brands voluntarily removed triclosan from their formulations in response to consumer concerns and shifting public perception. The World Health Organization and other health agencies acknowledge triclosan's effectiveness in oral care but recommend caution, especially given the availability of alternative ingredients that achieve similar results without the same environmental footprint.

Sodium lauryl sulfate, commonly abbreviated as SLS, is another ingredient that has become a standard in commercial toothpastes. It is primarily used as a surfactant, creating the foaming action people associate with "clean" teeth. While foaming does not enhance cleaning ability, it creates a sensory cue that convinces users the product is effective. From a manufacturing perspective, SLS is inexpensive and widely available, which explains its prevalence. However, research has raised questions about how this compound interacts with oral tissues and whether it is suitable for everyone. Studies show that SLS can be irritating to the delicate mucous membranes inside the mouth. For individuals prone to canker sores (aphthous ulcers), SLS-containing toothpaste has been linked to increased frequency and discomfort. Clinical trials comparing SLS-free and SLS-containing formulations have found that switching to an SLS-free product can reduce ulcer recurrence and improve comfort for sensitive individuals. The mechanism appears to involve SLS's ability to strip away the protective lipid layer of oral tissues, which increases susceptibility to irritation and inflammation.

Beyond sensitivity, there is also concern about how SLS affects the oral microbiome. While it is not an antibacterial agent in the same way triclosan is, SLS's detergent properties can disrupt the balance of beneficial bacteria. This may not pose a major issue for everyone, but in those with existing oral imbalances or conditions like dry mouth, its effects can be more noticeable. These considerations have led to growing interest in alternative surfactants derived from coconut or other plant sources, which create a milder foaming effect without the same irritant potential.

When evaluating fluoride, triclosan, and SLS together, the key is understanding context rather than approaching them with blanket approval or rejection. Fluoride remains a valuable tool for cavity prevention when used topically and in appropriate amounts, particularly for individuals at higher risk of decay. Triclosan, despite its demonstrated ability to reduce plaque and gingivitis, has largely fallen out of favor due to regulatory concerns and the availability of safer alternatives. SLS provides no direct oral health benefits beyond texture and foaming and may be best avoided by those with sensitive tissues or frequent mouth ulcers.

Making informed choices often comes down to personal priorities and health needs. Someone with frequent cavities might choose a fluoride toothpaste but opt for a formulation without SLS. Another person may prioritize botanical-based products and focus on remineralization through diet while using fluoride sparingly. What matters most is approaching oral care with awareness rather than habit, recognizing that marketing claims do not always reflect the full scope of scientific evidence.

This perspective allows for a more balanced relationship with modern oral care. Instead of feeling pressured to adopt every new "advanced" product, you can evaluate whether its benefits align with your health goals and whether simpler, gentler alternatives might serve you just as well. By blending evidence-based insights with respect for the body's natural systems, it becomes possible to create a routine that supports not only clean teeth but long-term balance and overall wellbeing.

Common Whitening and Mouthwash Ingredients That Disrupt Oral Balance

The pursuit of a bright smile and fresh breath has driven the oral care industry to create an array of whitening products and mouthwashes. While these products promise cosmetic improvements and quick fixes, many contain ingredients that can upset the delicate ecosystem of the mouth. What seems like a harmless rinse or whitening strip can, over time, weaken enamel, disrupt beneficial bacteria, and irritate soft tissues. Understanding the science behind these ingredients helps in making decisions that prioritize not just appearance, but lasting oral health.

Whitening Agents: Peroxide and Abrasives

Most whitening products rely on hydrogen peroxide or carbamide peroxide to bleach surface and subsurface stains. These agents break down pigmented molecules on the enamel, leading to visibly whiter teeth. Short-term use can be effective, especially for extrinsic stains caused by coffee, tea, or smoking. However, frequent or prolonged use raises concerns.

Peroxide is inherently reactive. While it lifts stains, it can also increase tooth sensitivity by penetrating enamel and affecting the underlying dentin. Research indicates that repeated exposure may lead to microscopic changes in enamel structure, making teeth more porous and potentially more susceptible to future staining or acid erosion. Although these changes are not catastrophic, they highlight the need for moderation and proper remineralization support alongside whitening.

Many whitening toothpastes use abrasives such as silica, baking soda, or even hydrated alumina to polish surface stains. Mild abrasives can help remove plaque and external discoloration, but higher abrasivity levels— often used in products marketed as "extra whitening"—can erode enamel over time. This erosion is gradual and often unnoticed until sensitivity or visible thinning appears. Enamel does not regenerate once worn away, which is why minimizing harsh abrasives is crucial, especially for those already dealing with sensitivity or gum recession.

Whitening Strips and pH Balance

Whitening strips, popular for their convenience, pose an additional consideration: pH. Some formulations are acidic, which enhances the bleaching effect but can temporarily soften enamel. If combined with acidic beverages or aggressive brushing, this softening can accelerate enamel wear. Neutral or slightly basic formulations are less problematic, but consumers rarely know the exact pH of over-the-counter products. This uncertainty underscores the importance of limiting use and pairing whitening treatments with remineralizing strategies, such as calcium-rich foods or topical products designed to restore mineral balance.

Mouthwash Ingredients: Alcohol and Antimicrobials

Mouthwash is often marketed as an essential step for fresh breath and germ control. The most common varieties rely on high concentrations of alcohol—sometimes exceeding 20 percent—to kill bacteria and create a strong antiseptic effect. While alcohol does reduce microbial load temporarily, it does so indiscriminately, eliminating both harmful and beneficial bacteria. This disruption can lead to rebound effects where opportunistic bacteria recolonize more aggressively, sometimes worsening bad breath rather than improving it in the long run.

Alcohol-based rinses also dry out oral tissues by reducing saliva production. Saliva is critical for maintaining pH balance, washing away food particles, and delivering minerals that protect enamel. A dry mouth environment favors the growth of acid-producing bacteria and increases the risk of cavities and gum irritation. For individuals already prone to dryness, whether from medications, stress, or mouth breathing, alcohol-based rinses can exacerbate the problem significantly.

Another commonly used ingredient in therapeutic mouthwashes is chlorhexidine. This antiseptic is highly effective at reducing plaque and gum inflammation, which is why it is often prescribed for short-term use after dental procedures or during active gum infections. However, chlorhexidine's strength is also its limitation. When used for more than a few weeks, it can disrupt the oral microbiome significantly, leading to staining of teeth and tongue, altered taste perception, and, in some cases, irritation of the soft tissues. Long-term reliance on chlorhexidine has also been associated with increased tartar formation, which counters one of the reasons people use it in the first place. Research supports its targeted use under professional supervision, but it is not suitable as a daily mouth rinse for those seeking balanced, preventive care.

Synthetic flavoring agents and sweeteners are also widespread in whitening products and mouthwashes. While they improve taste and user experience, some artificial sweeteners, such as saccharin or aspartame, can trigger sensitivities in certain individuals and may disrupt the natural feedback systems of taste and appetite. Synthetic dyes, commonly added to create appealing colors, offer no health benefit and can sometimes stain teeth or irritate sensitive tissues. These additives are rarely the direct cause of oral disease, but they contribute to a product environment focused more on aesthetics than on supporting the mouth's natural functions.

Many whitening and mouthwash formulations also incorporate stabilizers and preservatives designed to prolong shelf life and enhance product texture. Parabens and formaldehyde-releasing compounds are among the most scrutinized. While concentrations are typically low, cumulative exposure across multiple personal care products raises questions about long-term safety. For individuals seeking a cleaner oral care routine, minimizing unnecessary chemical exposure can reduce total burden on the body without compromising results, especially when gentler alternatives exist.

The most significant concern with many of these ingredients is their cumulative impact on the oral ecosystem. The mouth is not meant to be sterile; it functions optimally when beneficial and neutral bacteria coexist in balance with potentially harmful species. Overuse of strong antimicrobials, combined with harsh whitening agents and dehydrating alcohol, shifts this equilibrium, sometimes creating the very problems these products claim to solve. Rebound bad breath, heightened sensitivity, and recurring gum irritation are common signs of imbalance rather than a lack of cleanliness.

Supporting oral health without disrupting this balance requires a shift in perspective. Instead of focusing solely on cosmetic whiteness or the strongest antibacterial action, it is more effective to prioritize gentle cleansing, mineral support, and saliva-friendly environments. Options like alcohol-free mouthwashes with xylitol or herbal blends, mild whitening toothpastes using low-abrasion polishing agents, and short-term professional treatments for stubborn stains provide alternatives that respect the body's natural processes.

Choosing products with awareness means reading labels and questioning whether each ingredient serves a necessary purpose. Whitening and freshness are achievable without compromising long-term health when cosmetic goals are balanced with respect for the oral microbiome and enamel integrity. By combining a nutrient-dense diet, mindful daily habits, and selective product use, it becomes possible to maintain a bright, fresh smile that reflects true health rather than relying on quick fixes that quietly undermine it over time.

How to Detox Your Routine Without Sacrificing Effectiveness

Detoxing your oral care routine does not mean abandoning all modern products or returning to an era without toothbrushes or toothpaste. It means removing unnecessary chemicals, minimizing harsh ingredients, and creating habits that work with your body rather than against it. The goal is to simplify, not to compromise results. When you strip away what the mouth does not need, you create space for practices that strengthen enamel, balance bacteria, and support gum health naturally.

Begin with Awareness

The first step is understanding what is currently in your routine. Most people use products chosen out of habit or marketing influence rather than informed decision. Start by reading the labels on your toothpaste, mouthwash, and whitening products. Look for ingredients like sodium lauryl sulfate, triclosan, artificial dyes, and strong alcohols. These do not necessarily have to be eliminated immediately, but becoming aware of them allows you to make intentional choices rather than assuming they are essential.

Awareness also includes paying attention to how your mouth feels day to day. Persistent dryness, burning sensations, or increased sensitivity can all indicate that something in your routine is too harsh. Instead of ignoring these signals, treat them as feedback. Identifying which product or ingredient might be responsible helps you target adjustments without completely overhauling everything at once.

Gentle Substitution Instead of Elimination

Detoxing should feel like a process of upgrading, not depriving. Rather than removing every product overnight, start by replacing one item with a gentler alternative. Switching to a toothpaste free of harsh foaming agents or artificial sweeteners is often the easiest first step. Many natural toothpastes still contain fluoride for cavity protection but avoid unnecessary additives, making them a good transition for those not ready to go fully herbal.

For mouthwash, consider alcohol-free options that use xylitol, essential oils, or herbal extracts to freshen breath and support microbial balance. These alternatives avoid the drying effect of alcohol and are often suitable for daily use without disrupting the natural oral ecosystem. If whitening is part of your routine, explore low-abrasion formulations or short professional treatments rather than constant exposure to aggressive bleaching agents at home.

Focus on Supporting the Mouth's Natural Defenses

A detoxed routine shifts the emphasis from aggressive cleaning to supporting the body's built-in systems of protection. Saliva, for example, plays a central role in remineralizing enamel, neutralizing acids, and maintaining bacterial balance. Hydration, mineral-rich foods, and stress management all enhance salivary flow and composition, yet these aspects are rarely mentioned in conventional oral care advice.

Nutrient density is another overlooked factor. Vitamins D and K2, along with calcium and magnesium, are crucial for strong teeth and healthy gums. Integrating foods like leafy greens, pastured dairy, and fermented vegetables supports oral resilience from the inside out. This approach does not replace brushing and flossing but makes them more effective by giving the mouth what it needs to repair itself naturally.

Once you begin simplifying your products and focusing on supportive habits, the next step is creating a rhythm that is easy to maintain. A detoxed routine works best when it feels sustainable rather than extreme. Morning and evening care remain the anchors, but each step is chosen for purpose rather than habit. Gentle brushing with a soft-bristled brush and non-abrasive toothpaste, paired with thorough cleaning between teeth using floss or interdental brushes, forms the foundation. A simple rinse of salt water or an herbal infusion can follow, refreshing the mouth without stripping beneficial bacteria.

Whitening, if desired, can be approached strategically instead of daily. Short bursts of low-concentration whitening agents used occasionally, combined with polishing foods like crunchy vegetables and mineral-rich water, maintain brightness without constant exposure to bleaching chemicals. This not only preserves enamel but also helps shift the goal from unnaturally white teeth to a naturally clean, healthy look that reflects overall wellness.

Incorporating DIY options can further minimize reliance on additives. A basic saltwater rinse supports healing and balances pH after meals, while a rinse made from steeped herbs such as chamomile or peppermint can calm inflamed tissues and freshen breath naturally. These options are inexpensive, easy to prepare, and avoid preservatives common in commercial formulas. Baking soda, when used sparingly, can help neutralize acids and gently polish teeth without damaging enamel, particularly when combined with remineralizing foods in the diet.

Consistency is what transforms these practices from short-term adjustments into lasting results. Rather than adding more steps, focus on mastering a few simple ones and observing how your mouth responds. Over time, you may find less need for corrective products like harsh whitening strips or heavy antiseptic rinses because the foundation of balance reduces staining and bad breath at their source. The aim is not to do more but to create conditions where the body does much of the work itself.

Maintaining these results also involves awareness beyond brushing and rinsing. Staying hydrated throughout the day supports saliva production, which is central to oral health. Managing stress helps regulate cortisol, reducing its impact on gum inflammation and clenching habits. Even posture and breathing patterns play a role, as mouth breathing can dry tissues and shift the oral microbiome toward imbalance. When these lifestyle factors align with a simplified product routine, oral health becomes easier to sustain without constant intervention.

The greatest benefit of detoxing is the shift in perspective it fosters. Oral care stops feeling like a battle against bacteria and becomes an act of stewardship—working with the body rather than overpowering it. This mindset naturally reduces reliance on trends or aggressive marketing claims and fosters confidence in your own ability to maintain health with minimal, thoughtful tools. Over time, the simplicity of the routine becomes its strength, proving that effectiveness does not require complexity, only alignment with the body's natural rhythms and needs.

Part II. Rebuilding Oral Health Naturally

Having explored how modern habits and products have quietly undermined oral balance, it is time to shift focus toward renewal. Rebuilding oral health is not about starting over from scratch or adopting an entirely foreign lifestyle; it is about working with what you already have, restoring what has been depleted, and supporting the mouth's innate ability to heal. This part of the book takes you from understanding the roots of imbalance to actively creating conditions where teeth, gums, and the oral microbiome can thrive. The central idea here is that the body is designed to repair itself when given the right environment. Enamel may not regrow in the way bone does, but remineralization—the process by which minerals are redeposited into weakened areas of enamel—is constant and powerful when supported by proper nutrition and saliva. Gums, too, have remarkable regenerative potential. Even chronic irritation and low-grade inflammation can calm and reverse when harmful triggers are removed and nutrient support is prioritized.

Rebuilding naturally requires seeing the mouth as more than just isolated teeth. The gums, saliva, tongue, and microbiome function as a single ecosystem connected to the rest of the body. Every choice you make—what you eat, how you breathe, the products you use—affects this system either positively or negatively. This perspective helps shift oral care from reactive repairs to proactive nurturing, where prevention and healing happen simultaneously.

The chapters ahead will guide you through the pillars of this rebuilding process. You will learn how the oral microbiome can be restored to balance, why certain nutrients are indispensable for enamel and gum strength, and how traditional practices like oil pulling and herbal rinses complement modern science. You will also explore practical ways to reduce chronic inflammation, strengthen saliva's protective role, and design a daily routine that feels simple enough to maintain yet powerful enough to create visible change.

Most importantly, this part will empower you to rebuild without fear or overwhelm. Instead of feeling pressured to do everything perfectly, you will be equipped to make intentional, incremental changes that add up over time. By blending ancestral wisdom with research-backed insights, you will gain the clarity to choose what truly supports healing while avoiding extremes and unnecessary complexity. The result is not just a healthier mouth, but a stronger foundation for overall vitality—proof that oral health and whole-body health are inseparable.

Chapter 4: The Oral Healing Diet

Nutrients Your Teeth and Gums Can't Live Without (A, D, K2, Calcium, etc.)

Healthy teeth and gums are not simply the result of good brushing habits. They are living tissues, constantly breaking down and rebuilding. Every day, enamel loses minerals through exposure to acids and gains them back through a process called remineralization. Gums, meanwhile, depend on collagen integrity and a strong immune response to resist inflammation. Both processes rely on specific nutrients that work in synergy rather than isolation. Without them, even the most diligent cleaning routines cannot fully protect the mouth.

Vitamin A: The Foundation for Healthy Oral Tissues

Vitamin A is essential for the maintenance of epithelial tissues, which line the mouth and gums. It supports the production of saliva, a key component in balancing pH and delivering minerals to teeth. Deficiency in vitamin A can lead to dry mouth, delayed wound healing, and increased vulnerability to infections in the oral cavity. It also plays a role in the development of teeth during childhood, influencing the proper formation of enamel and dentin.

Food sources of vitamin A include liver, egg yolks, and full-fat dairy from grass-fed animals. Plant sources provide beta-carotene, which the body converts to vitamin A, though this conversion can be inefficient in some individuals. Incorporating a mix of animal and plant sources ensures adequate intake for tissue repair and salivary function.

Vitamin D: Regulator of Mineral Balance

Vitamin D functions as a hormonal signal that regulates calcium and phosphorus absorption. Without it, even a calcium-rich diet cannot effectively mineralize teeth or bone. Low vitamin D levels are linked to higher rates of cavities and periodontal disease, partly because of impaired immune responses in the gums and reduced density in the supporting jawbone.

Sunlight remains the most natural and efficient source of vitamin D, though dietary sources such as fatty fish, cod liver oil, and fortified foods contribute as well. For individuals with limited sun exposure, particularly during winter months, supplementation may be necessary, ideally guided by blood testing to avoid deficiency or excess. Adequate vitamin D not only strengthens teeth but also enhances the immune system's ability to manage oral bacteria without triggering excessive inflammation.

Vitamin K2: The Missing Link in Tooth Mineralization

Vitamin K2 is often overlooked in mainstream nutrition advice, yet it plays a critical role in directing calcium where it belongs—into bones and teeth—while keeping it out of soft tissues and arteries. This nutrient activates proteins such as osteocalcin, which binds calcium into the bone matrix, and matrix Gla protein, which prevents calcium deposition in places where it should not accumulate.

Research indicates that diets rich in K2 contribute to fewer cavities and stronger enamel, particularly when combined with vitamins A and D. Traditional diets provided K2 through foods like pastured egg yolks, aged cheeses, grass-fed butter, and fermented products such as natto. The scarcity of these foods in modern diets helps explain why oral and skeletal issues are increasingly common despite adequate calcium intake.

Calcium remains the most recognized mineral for tooth and bone health, yet its role is more complex than simply consuming large amounts of dairy. Calcium forms the primary structural component of enamel and dentin, but without adequate vitamin D and K2, the body cannot efficiently direct calcium into these tissues. This is why individuals with high calcium intake can still experience weak enamel or periodontal problems if these cofactors are lacking. The quality of calcium matters as well; sources from leafy greens, almonds, sesame seeds, and small bone-in fish like sardines often provide better bioavailability when combined with a varied, nutrient-dense diet.

Magnesium is equally critical but often underappreciated in discussions of oral health. It supports hundreds of enzymatic reactions, including those involved in bone mineralization and immune regulation. In the absence of sufficient magnesium, calcium cannot properly integrate into teeth and bone, leaving them more brittle over time. Magnesium also has a calming effect on muscle and nerve function, which may indirectly support oral health by reducing tension in the jaw and helping regulate nighttime clenching. Foods rich in magnesium include dark leafy greens, nuts, seeds, and whole grains, making it easy to incorporate through simple dietary choices rather than supplementation alone.

Trace minerals such as zinc and phosphorus, though needed in smaller amounts, also play vital roles. Zinc supports wound healing and immune function in the gums, while phosphorus contributes to the formation of hydroxyapatite, the crystalline structure that gives enamel its hardness. A balanced diet that includes whole grains, legumes, nuts, and quality animal proteins generally provides adequate levels of these trace minerals without the need for high-dose supplementation.

Supporting nutrients go beyond the obvious. Vitamin C, for instance, is essential for collagen synthesis, the protein framework that keeps gum tissue firm and resilient. Deficiency can manifest as bleeding gums or delayed healing after dental procedures, even when brushing and flossing habits are strong. Antioxidants found in colorful fruits and vegetables help reduce oxidative stress in the mouth, which is increasingly recognized as a contributing factor to gum disease. Omega-3 fatty acids from fatty fish or flax seeds also appear to moderate inflammation, creating a more balanced immune response to oral bacteria.

Integrating these nutrients into daily life is less about strict rules and more about building patterns that naturally meet the body's needs. Centering meals around whole foods—fresh produce, quality proteins, and healthy fats—ensures a wide range of vitamins and minerals without relying on fortified products or isolated supplements. When supplementation is necessary, it works best as part of a broader strategy that includes regular monitoring and alignment with dietary intake rather than as a replacement for nutrient-rich food.

The key is synergy. Vitamins A, D, and K2 work together to move calcium and magnesium into teeth and bone, while trace minerals and antioxidants maintain gum health and microbial balance. By understanding these interconnections, oral care becomes less about isolated nutrients and more about creating a nourishing environment where the mouth can thrive. Over time, this approach builds resilience—not just whiter or stronger teeth, but an entire system better equipped to resist decay, calm inflammation, and support overall vitality.

Foods That Promote Remineralization and Gum Repair

The health of teeth and gums is deeply influenced by what you eat every day. Beyond avoiding foods that harm oral balance, choosing foods that actively strengthen and repair is one of the most powerful ways to transform oral health from the inside out. Remineralization and gum repair depend on steady supplies of vitamins, minerals, and antioxidants, many of which are found in nutrient-dense whole foods rather than fortified products. When these nutrients work together, they not only repair microscopic enamel damage but also support healthy connective tissue in the gums and regulate inflammation throughout the mouth.

Mineral-Rich Foundations for Strong Enamel

Calcium, phosphorus, and magnesium form the structural foundation of enamel and dentin. Without these minerals, teeth cannot repair daily microscopic damage caused by acids from food or bacterial activity. Calcium is especially crucial, yet it must be paired with phosphorus to form hydroxyapatite, the mineral complex that gives enamel its hardness. Foods such as sardines with bones, yogurt, kefir, and leafy greens like collard greens or kale provide these minerals in forms the body readily absorbs.

Magnesium complements calcium by ensuring it is properly metabolized and deposited into bone and teeth rather than remaining in the bloodstream or soft tissues. Nuts, seeds, and whole grains are excellent sources of magnesium and can easily be incorporated into snacks or meals to support daily mineral needs. A balanced intake of these minerals is more effective than high doses of one alone, as they work in synergy to maintain tooth integrity.

Fat-Soluble Vitamins That Direct Minerals

Even with abundant minerals, remineralization cannot occur efficiently without fat-soluble vitamins, particularly A, D, and K2. Vitamin D enhances the absorption of calcium and phosphorus from food, while K2 directs these minerals into the proper places, preventing them from depositing in soft tissues and ensuring they strengthen teeth and bones. Vitamin A supports the development and repair of gum tissue and oral mucosa, preventing dryness and maintaining resilience against bacterial invasion.

Pasture-raised eggs, liver, grass-fed butter, and fatty fish like salmon provide these vitamins naturally. Fermented foods such as natto are particularly rich in K2, though aged cheeses and pastured dairy also contribute. Modern diets often fall short in these nutrients, which helps explain why even people with adequate calcium intake may still experience enamel weakness or gum issues. Prioritizing these foods restores the body's ability to direct minerals where they are most needed.

Antioxidants and Gum Repair

Gum tissue is highly vascular, meaning it responds quickly to changes in inflammation and oxidative stress. Antioxidant-rich foods help neutralize free radicals that damage gum cells and contribute to periodontal disease. Vitamin C is especially critical because it supports collagen synthesis, the protein framework that gives gums their structure and resilience. Without enough vitamin C, gums may bleed easily, heal slowly, or recede over time. Citrus fruits, berries, bell peppers, and leafy greens provide abundant vitamin C and other antioxidants that calm inflammation and protect gum tissue. Polyphenols found in green tea, pomegranates, and certain herbs like rosemary further enhance gum health by moderating bacterial activity and reducing plaque formation naturally. These foods not only repair but also create conditions less favorable for harmful microbes.

Protein is another critical element for oral repair, especially for gum health. Collagen, which forms the structural framework of gum tissue, is made from amino acids found abundantly in quality proteins. Without sufficient protein, even high levels of vitamins and minerals cannot fully rebuild connective tissue or maintain gum strength. Lean meats, fish, eggs, legumes, and bone broths provide the building blocks necessary for this regeneration. Bone broth, in particular, offers collagen, minerals, and gelatin in a highly bioavailable form that supports both enamel remineralization and gum elasticity.

Healthy fats play a dual role by delivering fat-soluble vitamins and moderating inflammation. Omega-3 fatty acids from fish like salmon, sardines, and mackerel have been shown to reduce markers of gum inflammation and improve periodontal outcomes in clinical studies. Plant-based sources such as flaxseeds and walnuts provide alpha-linolenic acid, which the body can partially convert to active omega-3 forms. Combining these fats with mineral-rich and antioxidant-rich foods enhances nutrient absorption and ensures that oral tissues receive the support they need for healing.

The way these foods are combined throughout the day can influence results. A meal featuring leafy greens, fatty fish, and fermented dairy provides minerals, omega-3 fats, and vitamins D and K2 in harmony, mimicking the nutrient synergy seen in traditional diets associated with strong teeth and broad dental arches. Pairing vitamin C–rich produce with iron-containing proteins improves absorption and supports collagen formation, directly benefiting gum tissue. Even snacks can be optimized by choosing mineral-dense options such as nuts and seeds paired with fresh fruit to balance acidity and promote saliva flow.

Timing also matters. Frequent grazing on carbohydrate-heavy foods keeps the mouth in an acidic state, which undermines remineralization. Consolidating meals and including fibrous foods that stimulate chewing helps restore a neutral pH and encourages saliva to deposit minerals back into enamel. Raw vegetables like carrots or celery, eaten at the end of a meal, can gently clean tooth surfaces while providing additional nutrients and fiber. This simple practice echoes ancestral eating patterns, where meals were less frequent and foods required more chewing, naturally supporting oral resilience.

Adapting these principles to a modern lifestyle does not require drastic changes. Starting the day with a breakfast that includes pastured eggs, leafy greens, and fermented vegetables sets a foundation of fat-soluble vitamins and antioxidants. Lunch built around wild-caught fish, whole grains, and fresh vegetables supplies minerals and omega-3 fats. Evening meals that incorporate bone broth, slow-cooked meats, or legumes with seasonal produce reinforce mineral and protein intake for overnight repair. By building meals around these nutrient-dense anchors, snacks and supplemental foods become optional rather than essential.

The shift toward remineralizing and gum-supportive foods is less about restriction and more about abundance—filling the plate with choices that work in harmony with the body's own repair mechanisms. Over time, these foods not only improve oral health but also enhance energy, immunity, and overall vitality. The benefits extend far beyond teeth and gums, reflecting the deep connection between nutrition and every system in the body. This approach transforms oral care from a reactive cycle of treatments into a proactive lifestyle that sustains long-term health and resilience.

Anti-Inflammatory Eating for Long-Term Oral and Systemic Health

Inflammation is both a friend and a foe. In small doses, it is part of the body's natural healing response, mobilizing immune cells to fight infection or repair injury. But when inflammation becomes chronic, it shifts from protective to destructive. In the mouth, this shows up as persistent gum swelling, bleeding, and tissue breakdown. Over time, low-grade inflammation does not stay local; it contributes to systemic problems ranging from cardiovascular disease to insulin resistance. Diet is one of the most powerful levers for reducing chronic inflammation and creating an internal environment where healing can occur naturally.

Why Diet Matters for Oral Inflammation

The tissues in the mouth are highly vascular, meaning nutrients and inflammatory mediators travel freely between the gums and the rest of the body. When the diet is rich in refined sugars, processed fats, and additives, it fuels systemic inflammation and disrupts the oral microbiome. This imbalance encourages the growth of harmful bacteria linked to gum disease and tooth decay. Conversely, nutrient-dense foods high in antioxidants, healthy fats, and phytonutrients help calm the immune system, strengthen oral tissues, and restore microbial balance.

Research consistently links dietary patterns to oral outcomes. People who follow anti-inflammatory diets—rich in vegetables, fruits, whole grains, and omega-3 fatty acids—tend to have healthier gums, lower plaque levels, and reduced markers of oxidative stress. These same patterns also lower the risk of heart disease, diabetes, and other chronic conditions closely connected to oral health, making them a foundational approach for whole-body wellness.

Key Nutritional Principles

An anti-inflammatory diet begins by prioritizing whole, unprocessed foods. Fresh vegetables and fruits supply antioxidants like vitamin C, flavonoids, and carotenoids that neutralize free radicals and support gum repair. Leafy greens, berries, and cruciferous vegetables like broccoli and kale are particularly potent. These foods also provide fiber, which supports stable blood sugar levels and feeds beneficial gut and oral bacteria.

Healthy fats play a critical role as well. Omega-3 fatty acids found in salmon, sardines, flaxseeds, and walnuts have been shown to reduce inflammatory markers and improve gum outcomes in clinical studies. Monounsaturated fats from olive oil and avocados provide additional anti-inflammatory support and help absorb fat-soluble vitamins crucial for oral health, including A, D, and K2.

Protein quality matters too. Choosing grass-fed meats, pastured eggs, and legumes ensures a steady supply of amino acids necessary for tissue repair without the pro-inflammatory compounds often found in processed meats. Bone broth and gelatin-rich cuts of meat contribute collagen-building nutrients that directly support gum structure and healing.

Equally important is the reduction of pro-inflammatory foods. Refined sugars, white flours, and industrial seed oils such as soybean and corn oil drive blood sugar spikes and oxidative stress, both of which fuel gum inflammation. Artificial additives and preservatives can also irritate the immune system and disrupt the oral microbiome. Reducing these inputs creates a cleaner internal environment that allows anti-inflammatory foods to work more effectively.

Building an anti-inflammatory plate can be done with simple combinations rather than complicated meal plans. A breakfast of leafy greens sautéed in olive oil alongside pastured eggs provides vitamins A and K2 paired with healthy fats that enhance absorption. Adding berries or citrus brings vitamin C and polyphenols that help neutralize oxidative stress. Lunch built around fatty fish like salmon with quinoa and steamed vegetables offers omega-3 fats, complete protein, and magnesium to support both gum health and systemic balance. Even dinner can reflect this principle: slow-cooked meats or legumes paired with roasted root vegetables and fermented foods like sauerkraut or kimchi provide minerals, antioxidants, and beneficial bacteria in one meal.

Snacking habits also influence inflammation. Frequent processed snacks spike blood sugar and maintain a state of immune activation, while nutrient-dense options stabilize energy and support saliva production. Nuts, seeds, and fresh fruit can satisfy hunger without creating acidic conditions that favor harmful bacteria. Chewing fibrous foods such as carrots or celery

63

between meals not only massages the gums and mechanically cleans teeth but also stimulates saliva flow, aiding remineralization and pH balance.

Hydration is another key factor often overlooked. Water helps maintain salivary flow, flushes food particles, and prevents the dryness that encourages pathogenic bacteria. Infusing water with slices of cucumber, mint, or berries can add antioxidants without the acidity or sugar of many flavored drinks. Green tea, rich in catechins, offers an additional anti-inflammatory boost and has been shown to reduce plaque formation while supporting gum health.

The timing and rhythm of eating also matter. Constant grazing keeps the mouth in an acidic state and limits the body's ability to return to balance. Structuring meals to allow periods of rest between them gives saliva time to remineralize enamel and reduces the inflammatory burden of frequent insulin spikes. This does not require rigid fasting but rather mindful spacing of meals and an awareness of how constant snacking impacts both oral and systemic health.

Transitioning to this style of eating does not mean perfection from day one. Small, consistent changes create lasting results. Swapping refined oils for olive oil, adding a serving of leafy greens to one meal each day, or replacing sugary beverages with water or unsweetened tea are achievable steps that cumulatively reduce inflammation. Over time, taste preferences shift, and foods that once seemed bland begin to reveal their natural flavors.

The greatest impact of anti-inflammatory eating is its dual benefit: as gum swelling reduces and oral microbiome balance improves, the same nutrients and compounds also support cardiovascular health, stable blood sugar, and stronger immunity. This interconnectedness reinforces why oral health cannot be separated from overall wellness. A diet that calms inflammation in the mouth inevitably benefits the entire body, and improvements in energy, digestion, and skin health often accompany healthier gums and stronger teeth. By embracing foods that work in harmony with the body's repair mechanisms, oral care becomes less about fighting problems and more about cultivating resilience that lasts for decades.

Chapter 5: Herbal and Natural Remedies for Teeth and Gums

Powerful Plant Allies: Neem, Clove, Myrrh, and More

Plants have supported human oral health for centuries, offering antimicrobial, anti-inflammatory, and healing properties long before the rise of modern dentistry. Many of these remedies have endured not only because of tradition but also because they work in ways that modern research now confirms. Neem, clove, and myrrh stand out as three of the most widely used plant allies, yet they are part of a larger group of botanicals that nurture the mouth's delicate ecosystem and assist in natural repair. Understanding how these plants function provides insight into why they have been trusted for generations and how they can be incorporated into a modern oral care routine.

Neem: The Bitter Protector

Neem, a tree native to India, has been a cornerstone of Ayurvedic oral care for thousands of years. Its twigs were traditionally used as chewing sticks to clean teeth and stimulate gums, and powdered neem bark or leaves were applied to treat infections. Modern studies validate many of these practices. Neem contains compounds such as nimbidin and azadirachtin, which exhibit strong antibacterial and antifungal activity. These compounds inhibit the growth of *Streptococcus mutans*—a primary culprit in tooth decay—as well as periodontal pathogens linked to gum disease.

Beyond its antimicrobial properties, neem also supports inflammation control. Its bioactive compounds help calm irritated gums and promote healing of minor sores. When used regularly, neem can reduce plaque formation and freshen breath naturally without disrupting beneficial bacteria. While bitter in taste, this quality is part of neem's therapeutic effect, stimulating saliva production and aiding in overall detoxification of the mouth.

Clove: Nature's Analgesic

Clove has long been used for toothaches and oral pain relief, a practice that continues in many cultures today. The key compound responsible for its numbing and antiseptic qualities is eugenol, which has been widely studied for its role in modern dentistry. Eugenol not only reduces pain but also possesses antibacterial and antioxidant properties, making clove a dual-purpose remedy for both symptom relief and underlying microbial control. Traditionally, clove oil was applied directly to an aching tooth or inflamed gums. In contemporary use, it appears in many herbal toothpastes and mouth rinses, often blended with other botanicals to enhance flavor and therapeutic effect. While clove is highly effective, it must be used carefully; concentrated clove oil can irritate mucous membranes if applied in excess. Diluted preparations or powders offer safer ways to harness its benefits for daily use.

Myrrh: The Healer of Tissues

Myrrh, a resin obtained from trees in the Commiphora genus, has a long history of medicinal use in the Middle East and North Africa. Revered in ancient healing practices, it was prized not only for its aromatic qualities but also for its ability to soothe inflammation and accelerate wound healing. In oral care, myrrh has been used to strengthen gums, reduce bleeding, and calm infections.

Research supports its antimicrobial and astringent properties, showing effectiveness against common oral pathogens and its ability to tone and tighten gum tissue. Myrrh also stimulates circulation in the gums, which enhances nutrient delivery and supports the repair of damaged tissue. This makes it particularly valuable for individuals with sensitive or receding gums seeking natural support in addition to conventional care.

Licorice root, though better known for its use in confectionery, has a long-standing role in traditional medicine for its soothing and antimicrobial properties. Certain compounds in licorice, particularly glycyrrhizin and licoricidin, demonstrate activity against cavity-causing bacteria and pathogens involved in gum disease. Unlike harsh antiseptics, licorice works gently, supporting balance rather than eradicating beneficial species. This makes it valuable in mouth rinses or powders aimed at calming irritation and promoting microbial harmony, especially for people with sensitive mouths or recurring inflammation.

Peppermint offers a different kind of support. Rich in menthol, it provides a cooling effect that soothes sore tissues and freshens breath naturally. Its antimicrobial activity is mild yet effective enough to discourage harmful bacteria without altering the overall oral microbiome. Peppermint's refreshing qualities also make it one of the most widely used flavors in natural oral care formulations, where it pairs well with more medicinal-tasting herbs like neem or myrrh, improving palatability without diminishing their benefits.

Sage, a herb deeply rooted in European and Mediterranean traditions, adds another layer of therapeutic potential. It contains rosmarinic acid and other compounds with antibacterial and anti-inflammatory effects, which help reduce plaque and calm irritated gums. Sage has historically been used in infusions or as a powder to massage gums, supporting both hygiene and circulation. Its gentle astringency can also help tighten gum tissue and reduce minor bleeding, making it a versatile option for daily maintenance.

Combining these plants often amplifies their benefits. A rinse made with neem, clove, and peppermint, for instance, can address microbial imbalance, soothe pain, and freshen breath in one preparation. Similarly, tooth powders blending myrrh and licorice can support gum repair while providing mild cleansing action. The synergy between botanicals arises not from a single active compound but from their complex mix of phytochemicals working together. This multifaceted approach is one reason traditional herbal remedies continue to hold value even as modern dentistry advances.

Incorporating these plants into daily routines can be as simple or as involved as desired. For those seeking convenience, natural toothpastes and mouth rinses featuring these ingredients are widely available. For a more hands-on approach, powders can be created at home by finely grinding dried neem, clove, or licorice and mixing with baking soda or clay for a gentle, remineralizing base. Herbal teas made with sage or peppermint can double as soothing rinses after cooling, providing both oral and digestive support.

It is important to remember that these botanicals complement, rather than replace, foundational oral care practices. They work best alongside regular brushing, flossing, and nutrient-dense eating, enhancing the body's natural defenses rather than serving as a stand-alone solution. Awareness of dosage and preparation is equally vital; concentrated oils like clove require proper dilution to avoid irritation, and certain herbs may not be appropriate for everyone in large amounts. Consulting with a knowledgeable practitioner or dentist familiar with integrative approaches ensures these remedies are used safely and effectively.

The continued relevance of these plant allies speaks to their adaptability and depth of action. They bridge the gap between ancestral knowledge and modern understanding, offering gentle yet potent tools for maintaining oral balance. By weaving them into daily routines thoughtfully and consistently, it becomes possible to support not just the appearance of healthy teeth and gums but the deeper vitality that true oral wellness reflects.

How to Create DIY Rinses, Pastes, and Poultices Safely

Making your own oral care products can feel empowering. It gives you full control over ingredients, lets you avoid unnecessary chemicals, and allows you to tailor formulas to your unique needs. At the same time, oral tissues are delicate, and the wrong proportions or ingredients can do more harm than good. Safe DIY approaches balance natural benefits with scientific understanding, ensuring that what you create supports healing rather than disrupting the mouth's ecosystem.

The Principles of Safe DIY Oral Care

The first principle is gentleness. The goal of any homemade rinse or paste is to assist the body's natural processes rather than overwhelm them. Many store-bought products rely on harsh antibacterials or high abrasives that strip beneficial bacteria or erode enamel. Homemade options, when prepared thoughtfully, can avoid these extremes by using mild yet effective ingredients like herbal infusions, mineral powders, and soothing oils.

The second principle is understanding purpose. A rinse for daily use should focus on balancing pH and freshening breath, while a poultice for irritated gums might prioritize anti-inflammatory and antimicrobial herbs. Each preparation should have a clear function rather than attempting to do everything at once. This clarity reduces the temptation to overload recipes with too many ingredients, which can increase the risk of irritation or imbalance.

The third principle is hygiene. Even natural ingredients can harbor bacteria or mold if not handled properly. Preparing small batches, using clean utensils, and storing products in airtight containers protects both effectiveness and safety. Water-based rinses should be refrigerated and used within a few days, while dry powders can last longer if kept in a cool, dry place away from sunlight.

DIY Mouth Rinses

Homemade rinses are among the easiest to prepare and use. A simple saltwater rinse remains one of the most effective tools for soothing irritation and supporting healing after dental procedures. Dissolving half a teaspoon of high-quality sea salt in a cup of warm water creates a gentle, mineral-rich solution that calms inflammation and helps neutralize acids. For daily use, adding mild herbal teas like chamomile or peppermint can enhance flavor and provide additional benefits without disrupting oral balance.

More advanced rinses can incorporate ingredients like xylitol, which naturally inhibits cavity-causing bacteria, or trace minerals like calcium and magnesium in liquid form to encourage remineralization. Essential oils such as clove or tea tree can be added in very small amounts for their antimicrobial effects, though they must be diluted properly to avoid burning or sensitivity. A single drop in a full cup of rinse is usually sufficient. Overconcentration is one of the most common mistakes in DIY oral care, and respecting the potency of natural oils is crucial for safety.

DIY Toothpastes and Powders

Creating a homemade paste or powder allows you to replace commercial formulas with mineral-rich blends that clean without harsh foaming agents. Baking soda is often used for its mild abrasiveness and alkalizing properties, helping neutralize acids and polish enamel gently. When combined with finely ground calcium carbonate or bentonite clay, it creates a base that supports remineralization while providing a smooth texture.

Flavor and therapeutic properties can be added with powdered herbs such as neem, clove, or licorice. These botanicals provide antimicrobial and anti-inflammatory effects while also enhancing taste. Small amounts of finely ground peppermint or spearmint can freshen breath naturally. If moisture is desired, coconut oil can be incorporated to form a paste, offering additional antibacterial properties and a soothing texture.

Poultices are less common in modern oral care but can be powerful when used correctly. They are applied directly to affected areas, allowing concentrated herbal compounds to work where they are needed most. A poultice made from powdered myrrh mixed with a few drops of warm water can soothe inflamed gums and promote circulation. For infections or persistent irritation, combining myrrh with powdered clove or licorice offers both antimicrobial and analgesic support. These applications are best used short term, such as during active flare-ups, rather than as part of daily maintenance.

When preparing poultices, texture matters. A mixture that is too dry will not adhere well to gum tissue, while one that is too wet may disperse quickly and lose potency. Achieving a paste-like consistency ensures contact without discomfort. It is also important to limit application time. Ten to fifteen minutes is usually enough to deliver therapeutic compounds without overwhelming sensitive tissues. Afterward, rinsing with plain water or a mild saltwater solution helps restore balance and prevents lingering residue.

Storage and shelf life are critical considerations for any DIY oral care preparation. Products that contain water or fresh ingredients should be made in small batches and used within a few days, as bacterial growth can occur even in the refrigerator. Dry blends, such as herbal powders for toothpaste or poultices, are more stable and can be stored for several weeks if kept in airtight glass containers away from heat and light. Clearly labeling jars with contents and preparation dates helps maintain safety and prevents confusion over freshness.

Frequency of use is another factor that ensures benefits without unintended harm. Even gentle ingredients can cause irritation if overused. Saltwater rinses can be used daily, but essential oil–based rinses are best limited to a few times per week. Clay-based tooth powders provide excellent cleaning but should be alternated with less abrasive options to avoid enamel wear in those with sensitive teeth. Listening to the body's feedback—watching for signs of dryness, tenderness, or changes in taste—provides guidance on when to scale back or adjust formulations.

Integrating these DIY methods with conventional care creates a balanced approach rather than an all-or-nothing mindset. Regular dental checkups, professional cleanings, and evidence-based treatments remain essential for monitoring oral health and addressing deeper concerns. DIY products excel as complementary tools, supporting daily balance, reducing inflammation, and extending the benefits of professional care between visits. This combination honors both tradition and science, using each where it serves best.

Ultimately, the safest and most effective DIY oral care routines are those built on simplicity. A handful of trusted ingredients—sea salt, baking soda, coconut oil, gentle clays, and a few well-chosen herbs—can meet most needs without the complexity of lengthy recipes or exotic components. By focusing on purpose, respecting proportions, and observing how the mouth responds, it becomes possible to craft rinses, pastes, and poultices that are not only safe but genuinely supportive of long-term oral health. This approach transforms home care into an intentional practice, rooted in awareness and respect for the body's natural capacity to heal.

When and How to Combine Natural Remedies with Professional Care

Natural oral care and professional dentistry are sometimes framed as opposing approaches, yet the most effective path lies in combining them. Each has strengths and limitations. Natural remedies excel at daily maintenance, prevention, and supporting the body's healing capacity. Professional care addresses structural problems, advanced disease, and interventions that cannot be achieved at home. Understanding when to lean on each side and how to blend them creates a comprehensive strategy for oral and overall health.

Knowing the Role of Natural Remedies

Natural remedies work best as supportive tools. Herbal rinses, mineral-rich pastes, and anti-inflammatory foods create an internal environment that promotes balance and resilience. They help prevent plaque buildup, soothe irritation, and encourage remineralization. This is especially valuable between dental visits, where consistent home care determines whether improvements hold or setbacks occur.

These remedies also empower individuals to take an active role in their health. Instead of viewing oral care as something dependent solely on professional cleanings or treatments, a person can cultivate habits that reduce reliance on invasive procedures over time. The goal is not to replace dentists but to minimize the frequency and intensity of interventions needed by maintaining healthy tissues and microbial balance naturally.

Understanding the Limits of DIY Care

While home-based approaches are powerful, they have boundaries. Severe decay, abscesses, advanced periodontal disease, and structural issues such as misalignment cannot be reversed with herbs or mineral powders alone. In these situations, delaying professional care in favor of solely natural remedies can worsen outcomes and lead to irreversible damage. Recognizing red flags—persistent pain, swelling, bleeding that does not resolve, loose teeth, or pus—is critical. These signs warrant prompt evaluation by a dental professional, as they often indicate deeper problems requiring targeted treatment.

Professional diagnostics also provide clarity that home care cannot. X-rays, periodontal charting, and clinical examinations reveal hidden cavities, bone loss, or infections that may not be visible or painful yet. Even those committed to natural care benefit from periodic assessments to ensure no silent issues are progressing unnoticed. Combining regular checkups with holistic maintenance prevents small concerns from escalating into major interventions.

Where Integration Creates the Greatest Benefit

One of the most effective ways to combine natural and professional care is during recovery and maintenance phases. After procedures like deep cleanings or extractions, natural remedies such as saltwater rinses, soothing herbal poultices, and anti-inflammatory foods can speed healing, reduce discomfort, and minimize reliance on pharmaceuticals. Similarly, between visits for orthodontic adjustments or periodontal maintenance, gentle rinses and nutrient-dense diets support tissue resilience and limit inflammation.

Integration is also valuable for prevention. Professional cleanings remove hardened deposits and reset the mouth's baseline, while natural methods help maintain that clean state. For individuals prone to recurrent issues, this combination offers a way to break the cycle of chronic irritation and repeated treatments. Over time, consistent natural care can reduce the frequency of professional interventions, though never fully eliminating their importance.

Clear communication with dental professionals is central to making integration work. Many people hesitate to mention their use of herbal rinses, oil pulling, or dietary changes, assuming these practices will be dismissed. In reality, most dentists appreciate being informed, as it helps them understand what patients are using and ensures there are no interactions with prescribed treatments. Sharing details openly allows adjustments where needed, such as pausing certain herbal remedies before surgery or confirming that mineral-based pastes will not interfere with fluoride treatments.

Choosing a practitioner who is open to integrative approaches can make this process even smoother. Holistically minded dentists or those familiar with functional medicine often have a broader perspective on prevention and may even recommend complementary strategies themselves. For those working with conventional dentists, framing natural care as supportive rather than as a replacement helps foster collaboration rather than conflict. Practical coordination also involves timing. Natural methods like oil pulling or herbal rinses are excellent for daily maintenance but should not replace antimicrobial rinses prescribed for short-term use after surgery or periodontal procedures. Instead, they can be reintroduced once the acute healing phase is complete to maintain balance without disrupting the treatment plan. Similarly, professional fluoride treatments can coexist with nutrient-dense diets and mineral-supportive rinses, each addressing different aspects of enamel health.

Preventive visits are an opportunity to refine home care routines rather than rely solely on cleanings to reset oral health. Asking specific questions during these appointments—about gum pocket depth, plaque levels, or areas of enamel weakness—turns professional checkups into personalized feedback sessions. This information can guide adjustments in diet, natural remedies, and brushing techniques between visits, making each follow-up more about progress than repair.

Addressing misconceptions is equally important. Some believe natural remedies eliminate the need for professional care entirely, while others assume professional treatments negate the benefits of herbal or mineral support. Both views miss the synergy possible when the two are combined. Professional interventions correct structural or acute problems, while natural methods sustain and amplify results, reducing the likelihood of recurrence.

The emotional aspect of this integration should not be overlooked. Many people drawn to natural care have had negative experiences with conventional dentistry, whether from discomfort, cost, or feeling unheard. A balanced approach offers reassurance that they are not abandoning their values while still accessing necessary professional expertise. Over time, this can restore trust in the process and create a sense of partnership rather than dependency.

Ultimately, combining natural and professional care shifts oral health from crisis management to continuous support. Natural remedies provide daily nourishment and balance, professional evaluations ensure nothing critical is missed, and together they create a cycle of prevention and repair that respects both tradition and modern science. This partnership does more than protect teeth and gums; it fosters overall wellbeing by acknowledging the deep connection between oral and systemic health and giving individuals tools to participate actively in their own healing.

Chapter 6: Oil Pulling, Tongue Cleaning, and Gum Massage

The Science and Tradition Behind Oil Pulling (Benefits, How-To, Timing)

Oil pulling is one of the oldest known oral health practices, with origins in Ayurvedic medicine dating back more than 3,000 years. In its earliest form, it was used not only to maintain oral cleanliness but also as a daily detoxifying ritual believed to influence the entire body. The traditional method involves swishing oil in the mouth for an extended period, allowing it to mix with saliva and interact with oral tissues. Over time, this simple practice has gained renewed interest as modern research begins to validate many of its observed benefits.

Historical Context and Traditional Use

In Ayurveda, oil pulling is called *kavala* or *gundusha*. It was prescribed as part of morning routines to remove impurities, strengthen the jaws, and prevent decay and gum disease. Oils used traditionally included sesame and sunflower, chosen for their warming properties and availability in India's climate. The practice was often paired with tongue scraping and nasal cleansing to create a holistic approach to daily detoxification. While early Ayurvedic texts framed oil pulling within a broader system of balancing bodily energies, the practical outcomes described—fresher breath, healthier gums, and reduced oral toxins—parallel modern observations.

Modern Scientific Insights

Recent studies have explored how oil pulling may influence oral health from a biochemical perspective. One of the most significant findings is its ability to reduce harmful bacteria in the mouth, particularly *Streptococcus mutans*, which plays a central role in tooth decay. Coconut oil, now widely used, contains lauric acid, known for its antimicrobial and anti-inflammatory properties. This fatty acid disrupts bacterial cell membranes, making it particularly effective against cavity-causing and gum disease–related microbes.

Research also suggests oil pulling can lower plaque scores and improve gum health when practiced consistently. While it is not a substitute for brushing and flossing, it appears to complement them by reaching areas that mechanical cleaning may miss and by altering the overall microbial balance toward a healthier state. Some studies have even observed improvements in markers of halitosis, likely due to the reduction of volatile sulfur compounds produced by oral bacteria.

Mechanism and Benefits

The process works partly through emulsification, where the oil mixes with saliva and creates a soapy-like solution that binds to debris, toxins, and bacteria. As this mixture is swished around, it penetrates crevices in the gums and between teeth. When spat out, it carries away these particles, leaving the mouth feeling cleaner and less inflamed. Regular practice can support a range of benefits: fewer cavities, calmer gums, reduced morning breath, and in some cases, less sensitivity.

Beyond oral health, some proponents claim systemic benefits, suggesting that reducing the bacterial load in the mouth lowers overall inflammation in the body. While scientific evidence for broader effects remains limited, the connection between oral and systemic health is well established, making it reasonable to view oil pulling as part of a larger preventive strategy rather than a cure-all.

Choosing the right oil makes a significant difference in both experience and results. Coconut oil is one of the most popular modern options due to its mild flavor and high lauric acid content, which has natural antibacterial properties. Sesame oil remains the traditional Ayurvedic choice and offers a warming quality that some find soothing, particularly in cooler seasons. Sunflower oil is another acceptable option and is lighter in texture for those sensitive to heavier oils. Whichever oil is chosen, it should be high quality, ideally cold-pressed and unrefined to preserve its beneficial compounds.

The method itself is simple but benefits from attention to detail. A teaspoon to a tablespoon of oil is placed in the mouth and gently swished between the teeth and around the gums. The key is to keep the motion light and continuous rather than forceful, as vigorous swishing can lead to jaw fatigue.

Ten to twenty minutes is considered optimal; this allows the oil to emulsify fully with saliva and bind to unwanted particles. Shorter sessions still provide benefit, especially for beginners, though longer durations may yield more noticeable results over time.

Timing also plays an important role. Oil pulling is best performed first thing in the morning on an empty stomach, before brushing or eating. Overnight, bacteria and metabolic byproducts accumulate in the mouth; pulling before breakfast removes these impurities before they are swallowed or reabsorbed. After the session, the oil should be spit into a trash bin rather than a sink, as it can solidify and clog plumbing. Rinsing thoroughly with warm water or saltwater afterward ensures any residue is cleared away and prepares the mouth for regular brushing and flossing.

Consistency is what transforms oil pulling from an occasional ritual into a meaningful part of oral care. Practicing several times a week is often enough for noticeable improvements in breath and gum comfort, while daily practice can enhance plaque control and reduce irritation. Results vary from person to person, depending on diet, existing oral health, and overall habits, but many people report fresher breath and cleaner-feeling teeth within a few weeks.

Safety considerations are straightforward but important. Oil pulling should never replace fundamental practices like brushing, flossing, and professional dental checkups. It is a complementary method rather than a standalone solution. Those with conditions like temporomandibular joint disorder should avoid prolonged swishing or use shorter sessions to prevent strain. Children under five are generally not suited for oil pulling due to the risk of swallowing oil, and individuals with nut or seed allergies must ensure their chosen oil is safe for them.

Integrating oil pulling with modern oral care creates a balanced routine. It pairs well with herbal rinses or mineral-based toothpastes, supporting gum health and microbial balance without harsh chemicals. Many find that starting the day with this quiet practice not only benefits their mouth but also sets a mindful tone, turning oral care into a moment of calm rather than a rushed chore. Over time, this combination of ancient wisdom and modern understanding offers a simple yet profound way to nurture both oral and overall health.

Tongue Scraping: Removing Toxins and Balancing the Microbiome

The surface of the tongue is one of the most overlooked areas in oral care, yet it harbors a dense population of bacteria, food debris, and dead cells. This buildup, often appearing as a whitish or yellowish coating, contributes not only to bad breath but also to imbalances in the oral microbiome. Tongue scraping, an ancient practice rooted in Ayurveda and other traditional systems, offers a simple yet powerful way to address this buildup and promote overall oral and systemic health.

Ancient Roots and Modern Validation

In Ayurvedic medicine, tongue scraping is known as *jihwa prakshalana*. It was considered a vital step in morning rituals to remove toxins that accumulate overnight. These toxins, referred to as *ama* in Ayurveda, were believed to hinder digestion and vitality if reabsorbed into the body. The practice was not merely cosmetic; it was seen as integral to balancing the body's energies and maintaining long-term wellness.

Modern research provides a different lens but confirms several of these benefits. Studies show that tongue scraping significantly reduces volatile sulfur compounds, the primary cause of halitosis. It also decreases bacterial load on the tongue's surface, which can indirectly reduce plaque formation on teeth and lower gum inflammation. While brushing the tongue with a toothbrush provides some benefit, scraping with a dedicated tool removes more debris and does so more efficiently without triggering the gag reflex as strongly.

Why Tongue Scraping Matters for the Microbiome

The oral microbiome is a complex ecosystem where balance matters more than total eradication of bacteria. Certain microbes on the tongue contribute to bad breath and gum disease, while others play a protective role, aiding in nitric oxide production and maintaining pH balance. When debris accumulates on the tongue, it fosters an environment where harmful bacteria dominate. Removing this layer through scraping helps restore equilibrium, allowing beneficial bacteria to thrive.

This balance has implications beyond the mouth. Oral bacteria influence systemic health through pathways involving digestion, inflammation, and even cardiovascular function. By reducing harmful bacterial load at its source, tongue scraping supports not only fresher breath but also a healthier environment for the body as a whole.

The Connection to Digestion and Taste

Another often-overlooked benefit of tongue scraping is its effect on taste perception. A coated tongue dulls taste buds, which can lead to stronger cravings for salt, sugar, or heavily spiced foods. Removing this layer restores the tongue's sensitivity, allowing for more nuanced enjoyment of food and potentially encouraging healthier dietary choices. Ayurvedic practitioners have long observed this link, viewing tongue scraping as a way to prepare the body for proper digestion each morning. Modern observations align with this, showing that cleaner taste buds can positively influence eating habits and satisfaction with meals.

Selecting the right tool is the first step to making tongue scraping both effective and comfortable. Traditional scrapers were often made of copper or stainless steel, materials still widely recommended today for their durability and ease of cleaning. Copper has natural antimicrobial properties, while stainless steel resists corrosion and is simple to sanitize. Plastic scrapers are also available and are lightweight, though they may wear out more quickly and are less sustainable over the long term. Regardless of material, the scraper should be smooth, with rounded edges to prevent discomfort or injury to the delicate surface of the tongue.

The technique is straightforward but benefits from mindful execution. After waking and before eating or drinking, extend the tongue and gently place the scraper toward the back, being careful not to go so far as to trigger a gag reflex. Using light pressure, draw the scraper forward along the tongue in a single motion, then rinse the tool under running water. Repeat this process several times, usually five to ten passes, until the coating is removed and the tongue appears clean. It is important not to scrape too aggressively, as excessive force can irritate the surface and damage taste buds. A gentle yet consistent routine produces the best results over time.

Frequency depends on individual needs. For most people, once daily in the morning is sufficient to remove overnight buildup and refresh the mouth.

Those dealing with chronic bad breath, heavy plaque, or digestive issues may benefit from an additional light scraping in the evening. However, more is not necessarily better; overuse can lead to soreness and disrupt the natural protective layer of the tongue. Observing the body's response and adjusting accordingly is the most sustainable approach.

Cleaning the scraper itself is part of the practice. After each use, rinse thoroughly with warm water and, if needed, mild soap. Periodic deep cleaning with boiling water or natural disinfectants such as diluted vinegar keeps the tool hygienic. Storing it in a clean, dry place rather than in a closed, damp container prevents bacterial growth and prolongs its lifespan.

Integrating tongue scraping into a broader oral care routine is simple. It pairs naturally with oil pulling for those who practice it, as scraping first clears debris and allows the oil to contact the tongue's surface more effectively. It also complements brushing and flossing, ideally performed afterward to ensure a fully refreshed mouth. Adding a mineral-rich rinse at the end can further support microbiome balance and enamel health.

The cumulative benefits become clear after a few weeks of consistent practice. Breath feels fresher throughout the day, taste perception sharpens, and morning coating becomes noticeably lighter. These improvements are not only cosmetic; they reflect meaningful shifts in oral ecology and reduced bacterial burden. Over time, these changes contribute to healthier gums, fewer cavities, and a more resilient immune response in the mouth.

By bringing together the wisdom of ancient traditions and insights from modern research, tongue scraping transforms from a simple mechanical act into a cornerstone of holistic oral care. It exemplifies how small, intentional practices can have profound effects when applied consistently, reinforcing the mouth's role as both a gateway and a guardian of overall health.

Gum Massage Techniques to Improve Circulation and Reduce Inflammation

Healthy gums are the foundation of strong teeth, yet they are often overlooked until problems arise. Bleeding, swelling, or tenderness usually signal inflammation, which if ignored can progress into periodontal disease and compromise overall oral health. Alongside proper brushing, flossing, and nutrition, gum massage is a simple yet powerful practice to improve circulation, calm inflammation, and support tissue repair. It draws from both ancient traditions and modern dental insights, bridging gentle manual techniques with a deeper understanding of how blood flow nourishes oral tissues.

Why Gum Massage Matters

The gums are highly vascular, meaning they rely on a steady supply of blood to deliver oxygen and nutrients. When circulation is poor, healing slows and inflammation lingers. Massaging the gums stimulates blood flow, promoting faster tissue repair and flushing out toxins that accumulate in stagnant areas. Improved circulation also supports immune defense, helping the body respond to bacterial challenges more effectively.

Another benefit is the mechanical stimulation itself. Light pressure on the gums encourages the production of collagen, the protein that gives gum tissue its structure and firmness. Over time, this can help reduce minor recession, tone the tissues, and restore resilience lost to chronic irritation. Gum massage can also ease tension in the jaw and facial muscles, which often tighten unconsciously due to stress or clenching habits.

Traditional Roots and Modern Research

Gum massage has roots in multiple healing systems. In Ayurveda, similar techniques are practiced using herbal oils like sesame or coconut to soothe and strengthen oral tissues. Traditional Chinese medicine also incorporates acupressure points around the mouth to influence overall vitality and organ health. While modern dentistry rarely discusses massage explicitly, research on tactile stimulation and microcirculation supports its value. Studies show that gentle mechanical pressure increases blood flow to gingival tissues and can reduce markers of inflammation when combined with consistent oral hygiene.

Preparing for Gum Massage

Clean hands are essential before beginning any oral massage. Washing thoroughly prevents introducing new bacteria to sensitive tissues. It is also helpful to rinse the mouth with water or a mild salt solution to clear away food particles and prepare the gums. Some people prefer applying a small amount of coconut or sesame oil to their fingertips for added glide and antimicrobial benefit, though this is optional and should be avoided by those with sensitivities to these oils.

Comfortable positioning enhances the experience. Sitting upright with shoulders relaxed allows easy access to the mouth without straining the neck. A mirror can be helpful for beginners to guide placement and observe technique, but with practice, the process becomes intuitive.

Basic Technique

Using the pads of clean fingers, gently press along the gum line in small circular motions. Start at the front teeth and move outward toward the molars, covering both upper and lower arches. Pressure should be firm enough to feel stimulation but never painful. If bleeding occurs beyond the first few sessions, it may indicate an underlying issue that requires professional evaluation rather than continued massage.

The goal is to stimulate, not irritate. Movements should remain smooth and steady, lasting one to two minutes per section. Breathing deeply during the massage helps relax facial muscles and enhances blood flow throughout the oral cavity. With consistency, this practice often results in gums that feel firmer, appear pinker, and respond less dramatically to everyday stressors like brushing or chewing.

For those comfortable with the basic technique, variations can enhance results by targeting different areas of the gums and jaw. Pinching gently along the gum margins between the thumb and forefinger provides a firmer stimulation than fingertip circles, which can be especially beneficial in areas prone to recession or chronic sensitivity. Another variation involves sweeping strokes upward on the lower gums and downward on the upper gums, following the natural direction of circulation toward the roots of the teeth. This directional approach encourages lymphatic drainage and may reduce puffiness or tenderness around inflamed areas.

Incorporating tools can also deepen the practice, though they must be chosen carefully. Soft rubber gum stimulators, often available in dental care aisles, are designed for massaging along the gum line without damaging tissue. Their angled tips can reach between teeth and around molars more easily than fingers. Wooden or metal tools, sometimes used in traditional practices, should only be considered if specifically designed for oral use and kept meticulously clean to avoid injury or contamination.

Adding herbal oils introduces another dimension of therapeutic benefit. Coconut oil provides mild antibacterial properties and a pleasant texture, while sesame oil, long used in Ayurveda, offers warming qualities that may soothe inflammation. Infused oils, such as those containing clove or peppermint, can further calm discomfort and freshen breath, though they must be diluted appropriately to avoid irritation. Applying a drop of oil to a fingertip before massage helps glide across the gum surface and delivers these plant compounds directly to the tissues.

Timing the practice for optimal benefit depends on personal routine and goals. Morning massage stimulates circulation after sleep and removes stagnation that accumulates overnight. Evening massage can serve as a calming ritual before bed, reducing tension from jaw clenching or daytime stress. Some people prefer to pair gum massage with oil pulling or after brushing, while others integrate it into moments of mindfulness, such as after meals when digestion begins. Consistency is more important than exact timing; daily or near-daily practice yields the best results.

Signs of improvement often appear gradually. Gums may look pinker and feel firmer, bleeding during brushing may lessen, and sensitivity to hot or cold foods can diminish. These shifts reflect better blood flow and reduced inflammation, not superficial changes. If discomfort worsens or swelling persists beyond two weeks, it is important to seek professional evaluation, as persistent inflammation can indicate underlying conditions requiring targeted care.

Integrating gum massage into an overall oral health plan amplifies its effects. When combined with nutrient-dense eating, regular brushing and flossing, and periodic professional cleanings, it becomes part of a comprehensive system that supports both immediate comfort and long-term resilience. This practice also fosters awareness; feeling the texture and tone of the gums regularly allows subtle changes to be noticed early, encouraging timely adjustments to diet, hygiene, or lifestyle.

Ultimately, gum massage is not just a technique but a way of reconnecting with the body's natural rhythms. It transforms oral care from a purely mechanical task into a mindful act of nourishment and self-maintenance. Through gentle, intentional touch, circulation improves, inflammation calms, and the foundation of oral health is strengthened, offering benefits that extend far beyond the mouth itself.

Part III. Oral Healing and Whole-Body Wellness

By now, it is clear that oral health is not an isolated concern but part of a much larger picture. The mouth is both gateway and mirror: what happens here reflects the state of the body, and what we put into the body is revealed in the mouth. Inflammation in the gums can echo inflammation in the gut. Mineral deficiencies that weaken enamel also affect bone density and energy levels. Even subtle imbalances in the oral microbiome can influence digestion, immunity, and cardiovascular health. Understanding these connections allows oral care to evolve from routine hygiene into a cornerstone of overall wellness.

This part of the book explores the bridge between local and systemic health. It shows how habits that support the mouth—balanced nutrition, mindful practices, and gentle natural remedies—also create ripple effects throughout the body. Conversely, it examines how chronic stress, hormonal changes, and environmental toxins manifest first in oral tissues, often long before they appear in blood tests or medical diagnoses. By recognizing these early signs, we gain the opportunity to address deeper imbalances before they escalate into more serious conditions.

The goal here is not to romanticize natural practices or reject modern medicine but to integrate the best of both. Traditional methods like oil pulling, herbal rinses, and gum massage align closely with what current research tells us about circulation, microbiome diversity, and immune regulation. When paired with professional evaluation and evidence-based treatments, they create a comprehensive approach that is both preventive and restorative. This holistic framework honors the body's innate ability to heal while staying grounded in safety and science.

Equally important is the shift in mindset that this integration brings. Oral care becomes less about fighting disease and more about cultivating health. Instead of reacting to cavities or gum problems after they appear, we begin to view every choice—what we eat, how we breathe, the products we use— as part of a continuous dialogue with the body. This shift fosters not only stronger teeth and gums but also deeper energy, clearer thinking, and resilience against chronic illness.

In the chapters that follow, we will explore practical strategies to harmonize oral healing with whole-body vitality. You will learn how the gut-mouth connection shapes immunity and inflammation, how stress and sleep affect everything from jaw tension to cavity risk, and how aligning daily routines with these insights transforms oral care into a powerful act of self-care. By weaving together science, tradition, and mindful practice, this section offers a roadmap for creating lasting wellness that begins in the mouth and radiates throughout the entire body.

Chapter 7: Stress, Sleep, and the Mouth–Body Connection

How Stress and Cortisol Affect Gums, Clenching, and Jaw Tension

Stress is often thought of as a mental or emotional burden, but its effects on the body are deeply physical. The mouth, in particular, reveals stress in ways many people overlook. Bleeding gums, chronic jaw tightness, and unconscious teeth grinding are not only dental problems but also signs of how the nervous system and stress hormones influence oral tissues. Understanding this connection allows us to approach gum and jaw health more holistically, addressing the root causes rather than only the symptoms.

The Stress Response and Cortisol

When the body perceives a threat, real or imagined, it activates the stress response. The adrenal glands release cortisol, often referred to as the stress hormone, to prepare the body for action. Cortisol increases blood sugar, heightens alertness, and shifts energy toward immediate survival rather than long-term repair. While this response is helpful in short bursts, chronic activation disrupts balance throughout the body, including in the mouth.

Elevated cortisol levels weaken the immune system's ability to fight bacteria in the gums. This makes it easier for plaque buildup to trigger inflammation and harder for tissues to heal once irritated. Cortisol also contributes to higher blood sugar levels in saliva, which fuels harmful bacteria and increases the risk of gum disease. Over time, this creates a cycle where stress not only exacerbates existing oral problems but can initiate them in otherwise healthy mouths.

Gum Health and Inflammation

The link between stress and gum disease has been demonstrated in multiple studies. People under chronic stress often exhibit higher rates of gingivitis and periodontitis, even when their oral hygiene routines are adequate. This is partly due to the immune suppression caused by cortisol, but stress also influences behavior: during periods of anxiety, many people brush less thoroughly, skip flossing, or rely on sugary snacks for comfort, all of which compound the problem.

Inflamed gums present as redness, swelling, and bleeding when brushing or flossing. Left unchecked, this inflammation can progress to deeper tissues, affecting the bone that supports the teeth. What begins as mild sensitivity can escalate into gum recession or tooth mobility, highlighting why addressing stress is as crucial as cleaning the teeth themselves.

Jaw Tension and Clenching

Another visible impact of stress on oral health is muscular. The jaw is one of the body's primary sites for holding tension. Under pressure, people often clench their teeth during the day or grind them at night, a condition known as bruxism. This unconscious habit places significant strain on the temporomandibular joint (TMJ), leading to headaches, facial soreness, and even tooth fractures over time.

Cortisol plays a role here as well. By keeping the body in a heightened state of alert, it signals muscles to stay contracted. The jaw, being part of the body's defensive posture, remains particularly prone to this tightness. Over weeks or months, constant clenching can create a feedback loop: tense muscles trigger discomfort, which in turn heightens stress levels, perpetuating the cycle.

Breaking the cycle of stress-related oral problems begins with addressing cortisol itself. Supporting the nervous system through lifestyle habits such as consistent sleep, mindful breathing, and balanced nutrition lowers baseline stress levels and allows the body to exit a constant fight-or-flight state. When cortisol levels stabilize, immune function improves, inflammation subsides, and tissues regain their natural ability to repair. Even modest changes, like pausing for slow, deep breaths before bed or choosing whole foods over refined snacks during stressful days, can reduce the biochemical load on the gums and jaw.

Physical interventions also provide relief for jaw tension and clenching. Gentle self-massage along the jawline, temples, and the area just below the ears can ease muscle tightness accumulated during the day. Applying warm compresses to these areas relaxes the muscles further, improving blood flow and reducing discomfort. Some people find relief from simple stretching exercises, such as slowly opening and closing the mouth or moving the jaw side to side, performed in a controlled and mindful way. These practices release stored tension and can prevent nighttime grinding from becoming as severe.

For those who experience bruxism while sleeping, protective measures like custom-fitted night guards help prevent tooth wear and reduce strain on the temporomandibular joint. These devices do not address the root cause but shield teeth and muscles from the mechanical damage of grinding. When paired with daytime stress management strategies, they create a comprehensive approach that protects both structure and function.

The connection between stress and gum inflammation also makes nutritional support particularly valuable. Diets rich in vitamin C, omega-3 fatty acids, and antioxidants strengthen gum tissue and counteract the oxidative stress triggered by cortisol. Leafy greens, fatty fish, citrus fruits, and berries provide these compounds naturally and complement the body's healing process. Adequate hydration further supports this by keeping saliva flowing, which buffers acids, washes away bacteria, and helps maintain a neutral pH in the mouth.

Mindfulness practices have an equally important role. Regular meditation, yoga, or even brief body scans throughout the day train the nervous system to recognize and release tension earlier. Over time, these practices help individuals become more aware of subtle clenching habits, such as pressing the tongue against the roof of the mouth or tensing the jaw during concentration. This awareness allows for immediate adjustments, breaking patterns before they cause lasting harm.

Professional support should never be overlooked. Dentists can identify early signs of stress-related damage, such as enamel wear or receding gums, long before symptoms become painful. Collaboration with healthcare providers also opens the door to referrals for physical therapy, counseling, or other integrative treatments that address both the physical and emotional aspects of chronic stress.

When approached consistently, the combination of stress reduction, nutritional support, mindful awareness, and professional guidance creates lasting resilience in both the gums and jaw. Rather than treating clenching or bleeding as isolated issues, this integrated approach acknowledges the deeper physiological patterns at play. As cortisol levels balance and tension eases, oral health improves not only in appearance but in its ability to support the rest of the body, reinforcing the profound connection between emotional wellbeing and physical vitality.

The Role of Sleep in Remineralization and Oral Repair

Sleep is one of the body's most powerful healing tools, yet its impact on oral health is rarely discussed. While most people associate sleep with mental restoration or general energy levels, it is also a critical period for repair processes in the mouth. The hours spent asleep determine how well teeth remineralize, how gums recover from daily stress, and how effectively the oral microbiome balances itself for the next day.

Nighttime as the Body's Repair Window

During deep sleep, the body shifts from active energy expenditure to maintenance and repair. Hormones such as growth hormone and melatonin rise, directing resources toward tissue rebuilding and immune regulation. For the mouth, this means microscopic cracks in enamel begin to remineralize, inflamed gums calm, and salivary flow adjusts to support healing. This nightly restoration is subtle but cumulative. Over weeks and months, the quality of sleep directly influences the resilience of teeth and the stability of gum tissues.

The process of remineralization relies on minerals like calcium and phosphate present in saliva. Throughout the day, acidic foods and bacterial activity deplete these minerals, softening enamel and creating tiny vulnerabilities. At night, when eating ceases and the mouth rests, saliva redistributes these minerals back into enamel. Deep sleep optimizes this process by supporting hormonal balance and allowing uninterrupted time for the minerals to integrate. Without adequate sleep, this restorative cycle is shortened or disrupted, leaving teeth more vulnerable to erosion and decay.

The Impact of Poor Sleep on Oral Health

Chronic sleep deprivation disrupts almost every aspect of oral repair. Insufficient sleep raises cortisol, the primary stress hormone, which can increase inflammation in gum tissue and slow healing. It also affects immune function, making it harder for the body to control harmful bacteria that contribute to cavities and periodontal disease. People who consistently get fewer than six hours of sleep often show higher rates of gum inflammation, slower recovery from dental procedures, and more frequent mouth infections.

Another consequence of poor sleep is altered salivary flow. Saliva naturally decreases at night, but when sleep quality is low or disrupted, this reduction becomes more pronounced, creating a dry environment where harmful bacteria thrive. Dry mouth not only increases cavity risk but also contributes to bad breath and discomfort upon waking. In severe cases, chronic dryness accelerates enamel wear and gum irritation, compounding other oral health challenges.

Sleep Disorders and Their Oral Effects

Conditions like sleep apnea further complicate the relationship between sleep and oral health. Sleep apnea involves repeated interruptions in breathing, often leading to mouth breathing throughout the night. This habit dries the oral tissues, disrupts the microbiome, and worsens enamel erosion by reducing the protective effects of saliva. It also contributes to jaw tension, as the body unconsciously struggles to maintain an open airway. Bruxism, or nighttime teeth grinding, is another sleep-related condition with significant oral consequences. Often linked to stress or airway obstruction, bruxism can fracture enamel, wear down tooth structure, and strain the jaw joints. It is both a sign of disrupted sleep and a contributor to further oral damage, creating a feedback loop that requires both dental and lifestyle interventions to address effectively.

Improving the quality of sleep begins with aligning daily rhythms to the body's natural clock. Consistent bedtimes and wake times help regulate hormonal cycles that influence oral repair. Growth hormone, which drives tissue regeneration, is released most abundantly during the deepest phases of sleep that occur early in the night. Missing these windows by staying up late can reduce the total time available for enamel remineralization and gum healing, even if total hours slept seem adequate.

Creating an environment that supports deep, uninterrupted sleep also enhances the restorative benefits for the mouth. A cool, dark room signals the body to produce melatonin, a hormone that not only aids sleep but also functions as an antioxidant, protecting oral tissues from oxidative stress. Reducing exposure to bright screens and stimulating activities in the hour before bed helps prepare the nervous system to transition from alertness to rest. Simple habits, like dimming lights and using quiet breathing techniques, set the stage for deeper sleep and more effective overnight oral recovery.

Nutrition throughout the day plays an equally important role. Adequate intake of calcium, phosphorus, and vitamin D provides the raw materials needed for remineralization. These nutrients do their work most effectively during sleep, when saliva redistributes minerals into enamel without interruption from eating or drinking. Avoiding heavy meals or sugary snacks close to bedtime further protects this process, as lingering food particles and acid exposure can interfere with the mouth's natural shift toward repair mode at night.

For individuals struggling with nighttime grinding or clenching, protective strategies safeguard teeth while addressing the root cause. Custom night guards, designed by dental professionals, cushion the enamel and reduce mechanical wear. Combining this with relaxation practices, such as gentle jaw stretches or mindfulness exercises before bed, addresses the muscle tension that often triggers grinding in the first place. When bruxism is linked to airway obstruction, seeking evaluation for conditions like sleep apnea is critical, as treating the underlying breathing issue often reduces grinding episodes and improves overall sleep quality.

Mouth breathing, whether from allergies, congestion, or structural factors, also undermines oral repair. Breathing through the mouth dries out tissues and reduces saliva's protective role in neutralizing acids and delivering minerals. Identifying and addressing the causes of mouth breathing—such as using nasal saline rinses, managing allergies, or consulting an ENT specialist—can dramatically improve the oral environment overnight. For some, gentle training techniques to encourage nasal breathing during the day carry over into better habits while asleep.

Recognizing the subtle ways sleep impacts oral health reframes bedtime routines as part of dental care rather than separate from it. Brushing and flossing remain essential, but pairing them with restorative sleep habits creates a foundation for lasting repair. Over time, the difference becomes tangible: less morning sensitivity, healthier gums, and enamel that resists everyday challenges more effectively.

When sleep quality improves, the benefits extend beyond the mouth. Reduced cortisol levels, steadier blood sugar, and enhanced immune function ripple through the entire body, reinforcing the deep connection between oral health and systemic wellbeing. Prioritizing restorative rest is therefore not just a lifestyle choice but a vital strategy for long-term resilience, transforming the simple act of sleep into one of the most powerful tools for healing and strengthening the mouth from within.

Breathing, Posture, and Relaxation Practices to Protect Oral Health

The health of the mouth is shaped not only by what we eat and how we clean our teeth but also by the way we breathe, the posture we hold, and the level of tension we carry throughout the day. These seemingly unrelated habits influence the oral environment, from saliva production to jaw alignment and even the development of cavities and gum issues. By understanding the connection between these everyday behaviors and oral health, we can take simple yet powerful steps to protect our teeth and gums over the long term.

The Impact of Breathing Patterns

Breathing through the nose is one of the most protective habits for oral health. Nasal breathing filters and humidifies air, supports nitric oxide production, and helps maintain proper oral pH. In contrast, habitual mouth breathing dries the oral tissues and reduces saliva flow. Saliva is essential for washing away bacteria, neutralizing acids, and delivering minerals that keep enamel strong. When the mouth stays dry for prolonged periods, bacteria multiply more easily, bad breath develops, and the risk of cavities and gum inflammation increases.

Mouth breathing also changes oral posture. The tongue often drops to the bottom of the mouth instead of resting against the palate, which can subtly affect jaw development and alignment over time. This is especially relevant for children but remains important for adults, as tongue posture influences the stability of the jaw and contributes to tension patterns that affect the entire face and neck.

Posture and Its Role in Jaw and Gum Health

Posture might seem unrelated to oral health, yet the alignment of the head, neck, and shoulders determines how the jaw rests and functions. When the head juts forward, a common result of prolonged screen use, the jaw is pulled out of its natural position. This adds strain to the temporomandibular joint (TMJ) and surrounding muscles, increasing the likelihood of clenching, grinding, and tension headaches. Poor posture also compresses the airway, making nasal breathing more difficult and encouraging mouth breathing during both day and night.

Maintaining proper posture supports both airway function and oral relaxation. A neutral head position, where the ears align with the shoulders and the chin is slightly tucked, allows the jaw to settle naturally. This reduces pressure on the TMJ and promotes balance between the tongue, lips, and teeth. Over time, these small adjustments decrease strain on the gums and enamel while also improving breathing efficiency and overall comfort.

Relaxation and the Oral Environment

Chronic stress directly affects the mouth through hormonal and muscular pathways. Elevated cortisol levels increase inflammation in the gums and impair their ability to repair. At the same time, stress activates the muscles of the jaw and face, often leading to unconscious clenching during the day or grinding at night. This combination of hormonal imbalance and muscle tension creates a cycle of irritation, recession, and enamel wear that no amount of brushing alone can resolve.

Relaxation techniques provide a practical way to interrupt this cycle. By calming the nervous system, these practices reduce cortisol, loosen jaw muscles, and restore healthy blood flow to the gums. Breath-focused exercises are particularly effective because they address both the physiological and psychological aspects of stress at once. Gentle nasal breathing, especially when extended into the lower diaphragm, triggers the body's parasympathetic response, signaling safety and allowing the jaw to relax naturally.

One of the most accessible ways to improve oral health through breathing is practicing conscious nasal breathing during daily activities. This can begin with simple observation, noticing when the mouth opens unconsciously and gently closing it while keeping the tongue resting on the roof of the mouth. Over time, this posture becomes natural and encourages proper muscle balance between the lips, cheeks, and jaw. Incorporating short nasal breathing sessions during breaks at work or before bed helps train the body to maintain this habit even during sleep, when mouth breathing often occurs unnoticed.

A structured exercise called diaphragmatic breathing is particularly beneficial. Sitting upright with shoulders relaxed, place one hand on the chest and the other on the abdomen. Inhale slowly through the nose, allowing the abdomen to expand while the chest remains still. Exhale through the nose in the same controlled manner. Practicing this for a few minutes daily lowers stress hormones, encourages relaxation of facial muscles, and promotes a steady flow of oxygen and nitric oxide, which supports vascular health in the gums. This method can also be combined with brief pauses at the top of the inhale and bottom of the exhale to deepen the calming effect on the nervous system.

Postural awareness throughout the day complements these breathing practices. Setting reminders to check alignment, especially during desk work, prevents the gradual forward tilt of the head that contributes to jaw strain and airway compression. Visualizing a string gently pulling the crown of the head upward can help lengthen the spine and reposition the shoulders without tension. Engaging core muscles lightly while sitting or standing stabilizes the torso and reduces the tendency to slouch, which often leads to clenching as the jaw compensates for misalignment. Over time, these micro-adjustments reduce the constant low-grade stress placed on the temporomandibular joint and surrounding tissues.

Relaxation techniques can be woven into daily routines without requiring long sessions. Simple progressive relaxation, where attention moves slowly from the crown of the head to the toes, consciously releasing tension in each area, brings awareness to the jaw and face. This awareness often reveals subtle clenching that persists throughout the day and offers an immediate opportunity to let it go. Warm compresses applied to the sides of the face or gentle circular massage near the jaw hinges further enhance blood flow and soften tight muscles, preparing the mouth for restful sleep and supporting overnight repair.

Even brief pauses to consciously relax the tongue can have profound effects. Resting the tongue lightly against the palate with the tip behind the upper front teeth creates an ideal oral posture that stabilizes the jaw and reduces unnecessary muscular effort. This position also supports nasal breathing and proper swallowing patterns, reinforcing the benefits gained from posture and relaxation work.

When these breathing, posture, and relaxation practices are applied consistently, the cumulative impact becomes clear. Jaw tension diminishes, gum inflammation eases, and the risk of habits like grinding and clenching decreases. The mouth feels more balanced and less fatigued, and the ripple effect extends beyond oral health, influencing energy levels, sleep quality, and overall resilience to stress. By integrating these subtle yet powerful habits, oral care evolves into a holistic practice that nurtures both the mouth and the entire body.

Chapter 8: The Gut–Mouth Axis

How Gut Dysbiosis Drives Cavities, Bad Breath, and Gum Disease

The connection between the gut and oral health is deeper than most people realize. The mouth is the gateway to the digestive system, and the balance of microbes in the gut profoundly influences what happens in the mouth. When the gut microbiome becomes imbalanced, a condition known as dysbiosis, its effects ripple outward, weakening oral defenses and creating an environment where cavities, gum disease, and persistent bad breath are far more likely to develop.

What Is Gut Dysbiosis?

Gut dysbiosis occurs when the natural community of bacteria, fungi, and other microorganisms in the intestines loses balance. Instead of a diverse ecosystem dominated by beneficial microbes, harmful or opportunistic species begin to thrive. This imbalance can stem from many factors: frequent antibiotic use, diets high in refined sugars and low in fiber, chronic stress, or inflammatory conditions like irritable bowel syndrome.

While dysbiosis is often discussed in relation to digestive symptoms such as bloating or irregularity, its influence extends far beyond the intestines. The gut microbiome communicates constantly with the immune system, hormonal pathways, and even the oral cavity. When this communication is disrupted, the mouth can become more susceptible to infections and inflammation.

The Immune System Link

A significant portion of the body's immune system resides in the gut. When the gut microbiome is balanced, it helps regulate immune responses, keeping inflammation in check. Dysbiosis disrupts this regulation, leading to chronic low-grade inflammation that affects tissues throughout the body, including the gums. Inflamed gums are more prone to bleeding, recession, and infection, setting the stage for periodontal disease.

This inflammatory state also affects saliva composition. Healthy saliva contains immune proteins and enzymes that naturally protect teeth and gums, but when the gut is imbalanced, these protective factors can decline. Saliva may become more acidic or less effective at neutralizing bacterial acids, weakening enamel and accelerating cavity formation.

Bad Breath and the Gut Connection

Persistent bad breath, or halitosis, is often blamed solely on poor oral hygiene, but gut dysbiosis is a hidden contributor. Certain gut bacteria produce volatile sulfur compounds and other metabolites that enter the bloodstream and eventually exhale through the lungs, creating an odor that cannot be resolved by brushing or mouthwash alone. In some cases, dysbiosis also contributes to acid reflux, which coats the throat and mouth with stomach acids and worsens odor while eroding enamel over time.

Nutrient Absorption and Oral Health

The gut plays a critical role in absorbing nutrients vital for oral health, including calcium, magnesium, vitamin D, and vitamin K2. Dysbiosis interferes with this absorption, leaving the body deficient even when dietary intake is adequate. Without these nutrients, enamel cannot properly remineralize, gums cannot repair effectively, and bones supporting the teeth may weaken over time. This creates a cascade where minor issues like sensitivity or mild bleeding progress into more significant oral diseases.

When harmful gut microbes dominate, they can influence the types of bacteria that thrive in the mouth. The oral microbiome and gut microbiome are connected by a continuous digestive tract, meaning bacterial imbalances in one area often mirror imbalances in the other. Dysbiosis in the gut can encourage a similar overgrowth of harmful oral bacteria, including species linked to cavities and gum disease. This explains why some people experience repeated dental problems despite careful brushing and flossing; the imbalance originates deeper than the mouth itself.

Research shows that certain inflammatory molecules produced in the gut circulate through the bloodstream and reach the gums. These molecules act like signals, triggering immune cells in oral tissues to stay in a heightened state of alert. Over time, this leads to chronic gum inflammation and accelerates tissue breakdown around the teeth. The process is slow but cumulative, and it often goes unnoticed until gum recession or tooth mobility becomes significant.

Cavities can also be traced back to nutrient disruptions caused by dysbiosis. Beneficial gut bacteria help synthesize and metabolize key nutrients like vitamin K2, which directs calcium to teeth and bones. Without this guidance, calcium may deposit in soft tissues instead of fortifying enamel, leaving teeth more vulnerable to acid erosion. A similar pattern occurs with vitamin D, which regulates calcium absorption and plays a role in immune defense. When dysbiosis interferes with these pathways, even a diet rich in minerals may not translate into strong, resilient teeth.

Restoring gut balance often produces improvements in oral health that seem almost indirect but are profound. As beneficial bacteria repopulate the intestines, systemic inflammation decreases and the immune system recalibrates. Saliva regains its protective qualities, gums heal more readily, and enamel benefits from better mineral availability. Breath freshness also improves as microbial byproducts decline and acid reflux stabilizes. The shift can be gradual, but many notice less morning dryness, reduced bleeding when flossing, and an overall cleaner feeling in the mouth.

Addressing gut dysbiosis requires a multifaceted approach centered on diet, stress reduction, and sometimes targeted supplementation. Increasing fiber intake from vegetables, fruits, and whole grains feeds beneficial gut bacteria, while reducing processed sugars limits fuel for harmful species. Fermented foods like yogurt, kefir, and sauerkraut introduce diverse probiotics that support gut balance. Hydration, regular movement, and mindful eating further enhance digestion and nutrient absorption, reinforcing the link between gut health and oral resilience.

Supporting the gut does not replace good oral hygiene but amplifies its effects. Brushing, flossing, and tongue cleaning remain essential for reducing local bacterial load, yet their benefits become more lasting when paired with systemic balance. A healthy gut equips the body with the nutrients and immune support it needs to maintain oral tissues, turning routine dental care into a more effective long-term strategy.

Recognizing the mouth and gut as partners in health shifts the focus from isolated symptom management to comprehensive healing. When both ecosystems are nurtured, cavities, bad breath, and gum disease become less frequent, and the entire body benefits from reduced inflammation and improved vitality. This integrated perspective transforms oral care into something far more impactful than a daily chore, highlighting its role in supporting the body's overall equilibrium and long-term wellness.

Probiotics and Prebiotics for Oral and Digestive Balance

The health of the mouth and the gut are deeply intertwined, and one of the most effective ways to support both is through probiotics and prebiotics. These beneficial substances help shape the microbial communities that protect teeth, gums, and the digestive system, influencing everything from cavity risk to inflammation levels. Understanding how they work, and how to incorporate them safely, offers a powerful foundation for oral and whole-body wellness.

What Are Probiotics and Prebiotics?

Probiotics are live microorganisms, typically strains of beneficial bacteria, that provide health benefits when consumed in adequate amounts. They help maintain balance in the microbiome, crowding out harmful bacteria and supporting immune function. While most people associate probiotics with gut health, research shows they also influence the oral microbiome, reducing harmful species linked to cavities, gum disease, and bad breath.

Prebiotics, on the other hand, are dietary fibers and compounds that feed beneficial bacteria. Unlike probiotics, which introduce new microbes, prebiotics nourish the ones already present, allowing them to flourish. By supporting this natural growth, prebiotics create a stable environment where both oral and gut microbiomes can maintain balance over time.

The Role of Probiotics in Oral Health

Specific probiotic strains have been studied for their effects on oral health. *Lactobacillus reuteri* has been shown to reduce gum inflammation and help control harmful bacteria responsible for periodontitis. *Streptococcus salivarius* strains, naturally found in the mouths of healthy individuals, can suppress bad-breath-causing bacteria and support a balanced oral environment. These probiotics do not replace brushing or flossing but act as an additional layer of defense, helping restore balance after disruptions like antibiotic use or high sugar intake.

Probiotic lozenges and chewable tablets are particularly useful for oral health because they allow beneficial bacteria to colonize directly in the mouth. Yogurt and kefir, while beneficial for the gut, primarily deliver probiotics to the intestines rather than the oral cavity. This means a combination of probiotic-rich foods and targeted supplements can provide the most comprehensive support for both mouth and gut.

The Role of Prebiotics in Supporting Microbial Balance

Prebiotics help beneficial bacteria thrive, ensuring they outcompete harmful species in both the gut and the mouth. Fibers such as inulin, found in foods like chicory root, garlic, and onions, serve as fuel for beneficial microbes. Polyphenols in berries, green tea, and cacao also act as prebiotics, enhancing microbial diversity and supporting anti-inflammatory pathways.

For oral health, prebiotics create conditions that favor protective bacteria over cavity-causing species. They can help maintain a neutral pH in the mouth, reducing acid erosion of enamel. In the gut, they improve digestion, enhance nutrient absorption, and indirectly support oral tissues by ensuring the body has adequate minerals and vitamins for repair and remineralization.

Combining probiotics and prebiotics creates what is often called a synbiotic effect, where beneficial bacteria not only enter the system but also find the nutrients they need to thrive. This partnership ensures that probiotics do not simply pass through the digestive tract but establish themselves in a way that supports lasting balance. In the mouth, this means helpful bacteria can colonize surfaces on the tongue, cheeks, and gums, preventing harmful species from taking hold. In the gut, it promotes long-term microbial diversity, which influences everything from nutrient absorption to immune resilience.

The most effective way to achieve this synergy is through diet. Foods like yogurt, kefir, kimchi, and sauerkraut provide living probiotic cultures, while high-fiber vegetables, fruits, and legumes supply prebiotics. Combining these in meals—such as pairing fermented foods with fiber-rich salads—creates a natural foundation for both oral and digestive health. Beyond whole foods, targeted supplements can fill gaps, especially during periods of stress, illness, or antibiotic use, when microbiome balance is most vulnerable.

When selecting probiotic supplements, paying attention to strain specificity is key. Not all probiotics serve the same function, and the strains beneficial for gut health are not always the ones most effective for oral care. For example, *Lactobacillus reuteri* and *Streptococcus salivarius* K12 are commonly studied for oral benefits, while *Bifidobacterium longum* and *Lactobacillus rhamnosus* are often used for gut balance. A formula that includes a variety of strains can support both ecosystems simultaneously, but dosage and delivery method also matter. Lozenges, powders, or chewable forms are better for oral colonization, while capsules designed to survive stomach acid are more suitable for gut targeting.

Prebiotic support should not be overlooked. While fiber-rich foods are the most natural source, supplements containing inulin or galactooligosaccharides can be helpful when dietary intake is insufficient. The goal is not excessive supplementation but steady nourishment of beneficial microbes. Too much prebiotic fiber too quickly can cause bloating or discomfort, so gradual increases and attention to the body's response are important. Pairing prebiotics with probiotics ensures a more stable and sustainable shift toward balance, rather than temporary changes that fade when supplementation stops.

Beyond diet and supplementation, lifestyle factors influence how well probiotics and prebiotics work. Chronic stress, poor sleep, and high sugar intake all disrupt the microbiome, no matter how many beneficial bacteria are consumed. Reducing refined sugar is particularly crucial for oral health, as harmful oral bacteria thrive on sugars and produce acids that erode enamel. Consistent hydration also supports both ecosystems, as saliva and digestive fluids rely on water to function optimally.

Over time, the effects of supporting microbial balance become evident. Fewer cavities, fresher breath, and healthier gums often coincide with improvements in digestion, energy levels, and overall resilience. These changes are subtle at first, but cumulative benefits emerge as the microbiome stabilizes and the immune system strengthens. Rather than addressing cavities or bad breath as isolated issues, nurturing probiotics and prebiotics creates a foundation of wellness that extends far beyond the mouth, influencing systemic health in profound ways.

By viewing the mouth and gut as parts of the same ecosystem, it becomes clear that caring for one always benefits the other. This perspective transforms daily habits—what we eat, how we supplement, and even how we manage stress—into tools for lasting oral and digestive vitality.

Healing Leaky Gut to Support Stronger Teeth and Gums

The gut lining is one of the body's most important barriers, selectively allowing nutrients to enter the bloodstream while keeping harmful substances contained within the digestive tract. When this lining becomes compromised, a condition often referred to as "leaky gut," microscopic particles of undigested food, bacteria, and toxins can slip through into the bloodstream. This triggers widespread inflammation and disrupts immune balance, with far-reaching effects on tissues throughout the body — including the mouth. Understanding how gut permeability affects teeth and gums offers a pathway to addressing oral problems at their root, rather than only managing symptoms at the surface.

What Is Leaky Gut and How Does It Affect Oral Health?

A healthy gut lining is made up of tightly connected cells that act like a selective filter. These cells allow vitamins, minerals, and amino acids to pass through while keeping out harmful compounds. In leaky gut, these tight junctions loosen. Causes can include chronic stress, processed foods, alcohol overuse, medications like nonsteroidal anti-inflammatory drugs, and persistent gut dysbiosis.

When the barrier is weakened, inflammatory molecules enter the bloodstream and circulate throughout the body. The immune system, detecting these molecules as threats, responds with heightened inflammation. In the mouth, this often appears as swollen or bleeding gums, increased sensitivity, and a greater tendency toward cavities and enamel erosion. The gums, which are highly vascular, are especially reactive to systemic inflammation, making them early indicators of deeper imbalances.

The Immune and Mineral Connection

One of the lesser-known impacts of leaky gut is how it disrupts nutrient absorption. A compromised gut lining absorbs fewer minerals and fat-soluble vitamins — including calcium, magnesium, vitamin D, and vitamin K2 — all of which are essential for maintaining strong teeth and healthy gums. Without adequate calcium and phosphorus, enamel cannot properly remineralize. Without vitamin D and K2, minerals fail to integrate into bone and tooth structures, leading to weaker support around the teeth and slower healing of gum tissues.

At the same time, chronic inflammation from leaky gut taxes the immune system, leaving it less able to manage bacterial populations in the mouth. This imbalance allows harmful oral bacteria to proliferate, contributing to gum disease and bad breath. In severe cases, the combination of nutrient deficiency and immune dysfunction can accelerate periodontal problems even when daily hygiene habits are consistent.

Early Signs to Watch For

Clues that leaky gut may be affecting oral health often appear subtly. Persistent gum inflammation that does not fully resolve with brushing and flossing, frequent cavities despite a low-sugar diet, or recurring mouth ulcers can all signal systemic imbalance. Other body-wide symptoms, such as bloating, fatigue, joint discomfort, or food sensitivities, often accompany these oral signs. Recognizing these patterns can guide a more holistic approach to healing, one that supports both gut integrity and oral resilience simultaneously.

Repairing the gut lining begins with removing irritants that perpetuate inflammation. Highly processed foods, refined sugars, and excessive alcohol are common triggers that disrupt the balance of gut bacteria and weaken the intestinal barrier. Replacing these with whole, nutrient-dense foods provides the raw materials needed for repair. Fresh vegetables, high-quality proteins, and healthy fats supply amino acids like glutamine, which serves as fuel for the cells of the gut lining, and zinc, which supports tissue regeneration and immune balance.

Reintroducing beneficial bacteria is equally important. Probiotic-rich foods such as kefir, sauerkraut, and yogurt help restore microbial diversity, reducing the dominance of harmful strains that contribute to gut permeability. Combining these with prebiotic fibers from foods like garlic, onions, and asparagus encourages beneficial bacteria to flourish, creating a more stable environment for healing. Over time, this improved microbial balance reduces systemic inflammation and indirectly supports healthier gums and enamel.

Key nutrients play a direct role in both gut and oral repair. Vitamin D regulates immune activity and enhances calcium absorption, while vitamin

K2 ensures that calcium is deposited in teeth and bones rather than soft tissues. Omega-3 fatty acids, found in fatty fish and flaxseeds, help calm chronic inflammation, making them valuable for both the gut barrier and gum tissue. Collagen or bone broth can also be supportive, as the amino acids they contain provide building blocks for connective tissues in both the digestive tract and periodontal structures.

Lifestyle factors exert a powerful influence on gut healing and, by extension, oral health. Chronic stress increases cortisol levels, which weaken gut integrity and elevate inflammation throughout the body. Incorporating daily practices such as mindful breathing, gentle movement, or even short walks after meals helps calm the stress response and improves digestion. Adequate sleep is equally vital; restorative rest allows the gut lining to repair overnight and helps regulate immune signaling that influences gum health.

Hydration, though often overlooked, is another cornerstone of this process. Water supports saliva production, which not only protects teeth but also begins digestion in the mouth, easing the burden on the gut. Proper hydration keeps mucous membranes moist and resilient, forming a first line of defense against harmful microbes in both the digestive tract and oral cavity.

As gut integrity improves, the effects become noticeable in the mouth. Gums that were once prone to bleeding or swelling begin to firm and regain a healthy color. Cavities form less frequently as nutrient absorption improves and enamel is better supported by calcium and phosphorus. Breath freshness often returns as both gut and oral microbiomes rebalance. These shifts happen gradually but signal a deeper harmony between the digestive system and oral tissues.

Healing leaky gut is not about following a temporary cleanse or restrictive plan but about creating a sustainable foundation. Prioritizing whole foods, balanced microbes, key nutrients, and supportive daily habits builds resilience that benefits the mouth and the entire body. In addressing the root causes of inflammation and nutrient depletion, this approach transforms oral care from surface-level management into a pathway toward long-term strength and vitality.

Chapter 9: The Impact of Hormones on Oral Health

Pregnancy, Menopause, and Hormonal Gum Sensitivity

Hormonal changes throughout life profoundly affect oral tissues, often in ways that go unnoticed until symptoms appear. Two major transitions, pregnancy and menopause, bring shifts in estrogen and progesterone that can increase gum sensitivity, inflammation, and even the risk of bone loss around teeth. Understanding these changes helps anticipate oral challenges, support healing, and protect long-term dental health during these pivotal stages.

How Hormones Influence Gum Health

The gums are rich in blood vessels and highly responsive to hormonal fluctuations. Estrogen and progesterone regulate blood flow, tissue metabolism, and the immune response. When their levels rise or fall sharply, the gums often react with increased sensitivity and inflammation. This does not mean that hormonal changes directly cause gum disease, but they can magnify the body's reaction to plaque and other irritants. What might have been minor irritation in a stable hormonal state can escalate into significant swelling or bleeding during periods of hormonal transition.

Pregnancy and Oral Changes

Pregnancy brings dramatic increases in estrogen and progesterone to support fetal development. These hormones enhance blood flow to the gums, making them more prone to swelling and tenderness. Many women experience "pregnancy gingivitis," marked by red, sensitive gums that bleed easily during brushing or flossing. This condition can begin as early as the second month and may peak during the second trimester.

In addition to increased blood flow, hormonal changes alter the way the immune system responds to bacteria. The body shifts toward a state of immune tolerance to protect the developing fetus, which can also reduce resistance to oral pathogens. As a result, plaque buildup triggers stronger inflammatory reactions, leading to discomfort and heightened risk of gum disease if oral hygiene is not carefully maintained.

Pregnancy can also bring changes in saliva composition and pH. Morning sickness and acid reflux expose teeth to stomach acids, weakening enamel and raising cavity risk. Cravings for carbohydrates or increased snacking may add to this challenge, feeding acid-producing bacteria in the mouth. Together, these factors make consistent oral care during pregnancy not only safe but essential.

Menopause and the Oral Microenvironment

Menopause introduces a different hormonal challenge: declining estrogen levels. Estrogen helps maintain bone density, including the jawbone that supports teeth. As levels fall, bone may gradually thin, increasing the risk of tooth mobility and gum recession. Lower estrogen also reduces saliva production, contributing to dry mouth, which fosters bacterial overgrowth and accelerates decay.

Gum tissues themselves can become thinner and less resilient after menopause, making them more susceptible to irritation from plaque or dental appliances. Burning mouth syndrome, a condition marked by chronic oral discomfort without visible lesions, is also more common in postmenopausal women and is thought to be linked to both hormonal and nervous system changes.

Supporting gum health during these hormonal shifts begins with consistency in oral hygiene. Gentle but thorough brushing with a soft-bristled toothbrush twice daily removes plaque without aggravating already sensitive gums. Flossing remains important, though it may need to be done more carefully if bleeding is frequent. In some cases, switching to water flossers can help reduce discomfort while still maintaining gum cleanliness. Using a mild, alcohol-free rinse can soothe inflammation and reduce bacterial buildup without further irritating tissues.

Nutrition plays a critical role in protecting both teeth and gums during these transitions. Adequate intake of calcium, vitamin D, and vitamin K2 supports the remineralization of enamel and strengthens the bone structure underlying the teeth. Vitamin C is equally important for collagen production, which helps maintain gum integrity and aids in healing microtears caused by inflammation. For pregnant women, incorporating

112

folate-rich foods like leafy greens supports both fetal development and gum health, as folate deficiency has been linked to periodontal issues. Staying hydrated is also vital, especially during menopause when dry mouth becomes more common. Sufficient water intake helps maintain saliva flow, which naturally buffers acids and carries minerals to the teeth.

Managing inflammation through diet can provide additional relief. Omega-3 fatty acids from sources like fatty fish, chia seeds, or flaxseeds reduce inflammatory markers and support gum healing. Limiting processed sugars and refined carbohydrates is equally important, as these foods feed harmful bacteria and promote plaque buildup. For women experiencing frequent reflux during pregnancy, minimizing acidic foods and avoiding eating right before bedtime can help reduce enamel erosion and gum irritation caused by stomach acids.

Regular professional dental care becomes even more valuable during pregnancy and menopause. Cleanings every three to four months, rather than the standard six, can help manage the increased plaque accumulation and gum sensitivity common during these stages. Dental professionals can also identify early changes in gum health, bone density, or enamel integrity, allowing for timely interventions that prevent more serious problems later. Routine checkups are considered safe during pregnancy, and many dentists recommend scheduling a cleaning in the second trimester when gum inflammation tends to peak.

Addressing dry mouth, particularly in menopause, may involve simple adjustments such as sipping water frequently, chewing sugar-free xylitol gum to stimulate saliva, or using saliva-enhancing rinses. Avoiding mouthwashes with alcohol and limiting caffeine intake also help prevent further dryness. For those experiencing burning mouth syndrome or heightened oral discomfort, consulting a dental professional familiar with menopausal symptoms can guide tailored approaches, from nutritional support to specific topical treatments.

Stress management is another overlooked factor that influences hormonal and oral health alike. Chronic stress elevates cortisol levels, which can worsen gum inflammation and slow tissue repair. Gentle relaxation techniques, such as diaphragmatic breathing or restorative yoga, help regulate stress hormones and indirectly protect oral tissues. Adequate sleep further enhances immune function and supports both hormonal and oral balance, reinforcing the benefits of other lifestyle strategies.

By approaching gum sensitivity during pregnancy and menopause with a combination of consistent hygiene, targeted nutrition, professional support, and mindful lifestyle choices, it is possible to navigate these transitions with resilience. Instead of viewing hormonal changes as inevitable pathways to oral decline, they can become opportunities to deepen awareness of the body's needs and build habits that safeguard teeth and gums well into later life.

Blood Sugar, Insulin Resistance, and Tooth Decay

The link between blood sugar control and oral health is stronger than many people realize. While cavities are often associated with sugar consumption alone, the body's ability to process that sugar plays an equally important role. Chronic blood sugar imbalances and insulin resistance do more than increase cavity risk; they alter saliva composition, fuel harmful bacterial growth, and impair the gums' capacity to repair themselves. Understanding how metabolic health shapes oral health offers insight into why dental problems are sometimes a symptom of deeper systemic issues.

How Blood Sugar Affects the Mouth

When blood sugar levels remain consistently high, as in prediabetes or diabetes, the mouth becomes more vulnerable to decay and inflammation. Elevated glucose appears in saliva, providing an ideal food source for cavity-causing bacteria such as *Streptococcus mutans*. These bacteria metabolize sugars into acids that erode enamel and irritate gum tissue. Over time, the cycle of high sugar and acid exposure weakens teeth and leaves them prone to cavities, even in individuals who maintain good brushing habits.

High blood sugar also affects the immune response within the mouth. White blood cells become less efficient at controlling bacterial populations, making gum disease more likely and harder to manage. This combination of increased bacterial growth and reduced immune defense accelerates the progression of periodontal disease, leading to gum recession and potential tooth loss if left unaddressed.

Insulin Resistance and Oral Health

Insulin resistance, often a precursor to type 2 diabetes, intensifies these risks by disrupting the body's ability to regulate glucose effectively. When cells become less responsive to insulin, blood sugar remains elevated for longer periods after meals. This prolonged exposure allows harmful oral bacteria more time to feed and produce acids that damage enamel.

Insulin resistance is also associated with chronic low-grade inflammation, which affects the gums and underlying bone structure. Inflammatory markers rise throughout the body, including in the tissues that support teeth, making them more susceptible to infection and slower to heal. This is one reason why people with metabolic syndrome often experience more severe gum disease and require more intensive dental care.

The Role of Saliva and pH Balance

Blood sugar imbalances influence not only the presence of bacteria but also the quality of saliva. Healthy saliva naturally buffers acids, provides minerals like calcium and phosphate for enamel repair, and washes away food particles. In individuals with poorly controlled blood sugar, saliva often becomes thicker and less effective at neutralizing acids, leaving teeth more exposed to erosion. Additionally, frequent dry mouth, common in people with diabetes, exacerbates these effects and contributes to bad breath.

The mouth's pH level also shifts under chronic high sugar conditions. Acidic environments favor the growth of harmful bacteria while inhibiting beneficial species that protect against decay. This imbalance in the oral microbiome creates a vicious cycle, where acid-producing bacteria dominate and beneficial bacteria struggle to regain control.

Balancing blood sugar begins with dietary choices that minimize rapid spikes and crashes. Emphasizing whole foods with a low glycemic load helps reduce the constant feed of glucose that fuels harmful oral bacteria. Meals centered on vegetables, lean proteins, healthy fats, and fiber-rich carbohydrates provide steady energy and help maintain stable insulin levels. Avoiding frequent snacking on sugary or refined foods reduces the number of acid attacks on enamel and gives saliva time to restore a neutral pH between meals.

Nutrient intake plays a crucial role in repairing and protecting oral tissues affected by high blood sugar. Magnesium and chromium support insulin sensitivity, allowing the body to use glucose more effectively and lowering the risk of persistent hyperglycemia that damages teeth and gums. Vitamin D enhances calcium absorption and strengthens both enamel and the bone surrounding the teeth. Omega-3 fatty acids reduce systemic inflammation, indirectly calming inflamed gum tissue and improving healing outcomes. Prioritizing these nutrients through diet, and supplementing when necessary under professional guidance, supports both metabolic and oral resilience.

Physical activity is another critical factor in improving insulin sensitivity and protecting oral health. Regular exercise helps muscles absorb glucose more efficiently, reducing the time that elevated blood sugar lingers after meals.

Even moderate activities such as walking after eating can blunt post-meal spikes and lower overall inflammation levels. This metabolic improvement translates into a healthier oral environment, where saliva composition normalizes and gum tissues regain their ability to repair microdamage more effectively.

Stress management complements these physical strategies. Chronic stress elevates cortisol, which not only raises blood sugar but also suppresses immune defenses in the mouth. Integrating breathing exercises, meditation, or gentle movement practices like yoga reduces cortisol and supports better glycemic control. As stress diminishes, the body can redirect energy toward healing and maintaining gum health rather than constantly responding to perceived threats.

Oral hygiene practices remain essential, but they become even more effective when paired with improved blood sugar control. Brushing twice daily with fluoride or hydroxyapatite toothpaste protects enamel from acid erosion, while flossing and tongue cleaning help manage bacterial buildup that thrives on excess sugars. For individuals with persistent dry mouth, sipping water regularly and using xylitol-containing gums or lozenges can stimulate saliva production, restoring the mouth's natural defense against cavities and acidity.

Professional dental care plays a preventive role as well. More frequent cleanings and checkups may be recommended for individuals with blood sugar challenges to monitor gum health and catch early signs of decay or infection. Dentists can also provide guidance on managing dry mouth, identifying enamel erosion from acidic conditions, and coordinating care with medical professionals who oversee metabolic conditions.

Improving blood sugar and insulin sensitivity does more than protect teeth and gums; it supports whole-body health. As glucose levels stabilize, inflammation throughout the body decreases, energy levels rise, and the immune system functions more effectively. This systemic improvement creates a feedback loop where oral health further supports metabolic health, since chronic gum inflammation has been shown to worsen insulin resistance. Addressing both simultaneously transforms dental care from a reactive process into a proactive strategy for long-term wellness.

By viewing tooth decay and gum disease through the lens of blood sugar regulation, prevention shifts from merely avoiding sweets to cultivating metabolic balance. This broader approach empowers individuals to not only safeguard their oral health but also improve cardiovascular, hormonal, and overall well-being, making the care of teeth and gums an integral part of a much larger picture of health.

Supporting Hormonal Balance for Lifelong Oral Resilience

Hormones influence nearly every aspect of oral health, from the way gums respond to bacteria to how bones around the teeth maintain their strength. Fluctuations in estrogen, progesterone, cortisol, thyroid hormones, and insulin can either strengthen or weaken the oral environment depending on their balance. While life stages such as puberty, pregnancy, and menopause bring predictable hormonal shifts, everyday habits, stress, and diet also play a powerful role in shaping hormonal patterns. Learning to support hormonal balance is therefore not only key to overall health but also essential for protecting teeth and gums throughout life.

The Hormone–Oral Health Connection

The gums and jawbone are highly sensitive to changes in hormone levels. Estrogen helps maintain the density of the alveolar bone that anchors teeth, while progesterone influences blood flow and inflammation in gum tissues. Cortisol, the body's primary stress hormone, directly affects immune function and inflammation, often increasing gum sensitivity when chronically elevated. Insulin regulates blood sugar, which in turn determines how much fuel oral bacteria have to produce acids that erode enamel. When these hormones are in harmony, the mouth is better able to resist plaque, heal after minor injuries, and recover from inflammation.

Disruptions in hormonal balance, however, create vulnerabilities. Elevated cortisol from chronic stress can increase inflammation and delay gum healing. Insulin resistance fuels bacterial growth and worsens acid exposure on enamel. Declining estrogen during menopause contributes to dry mouth and bone loss, heightening the risk of periodontal disease and tooth mobility. Even subtle hormonal shifts, such as those caused by lack of sleep or erratic eating patterns, can accumulate over time and impact oral resilience.

Nutrition for Hormonal and Oral Support

Food choices are central to balancing hormones and protecting oral tissues. Stable blood sugar is one of the most powerful levers, as frequent spikes from refined sugars and processed carbohydrates disrupt insulin regulation

119

and feed harmful oral bacteria. Prioritizing whole foods rich in fiber, protein, and healthy fats helps maintain steady energy and reduces inflammatory swings that strain the gums and jawbone.

Micronutrients play an equally vital role. Magnesium supports hundreds of enzymatic processes, including those that regulate stress response and blood sugar. Vitamin D not only enhances calcium absorption for strong enamel and bone but also influences immune function, lowering the likelihood of gum inflammation. Vitamin K2 directs calcium to teeth and bones rather than soft tissues, while omega-3 fatty acids help modulate inflammation throughout the body, including the mouth. Together, these nutrients form the biochemical foundation for both hormonal equilibrium and oral repair.

The Role of Lifestyle and Stress Management

Hormonal health is deeply tied to daily rhythms. Chronic stress, irregular sleep, and a sedentary lifestyle disrupt cortisol patterns and throw other hormones out of balance. Elevated cortisol increases inflammation in the gums and can contribute to nighttime clenching or grinding. Lack of restorative sleep interferes with growth hormone release, a key player in tissue repair, and disrupts insulin sensitivity, further compounding blood sugar fluctuations.

Incorporating simple stress-reducing practices has direct benefits for oral health. Breath-based relaxation, walking outdoors, and mindfulness exercises lower cortisol and create more favorable conditions for healing tissues and maintaining microbial balance. Adequate sleep, ideally aligned with natural light cycles, allows the body to perform nightly maintenance that benefits the gums and jaw as much as the rest of the body.

Adapting care strategies to different life stages ensures that hormonal shifts do not undermine oral health. During puberty and pregnancy, when estrogen and progesterone rise, gums can become more sensitive and reactive to plaque. This is often the first time individuals notice gum bleeding despite consistent brushing. Increasing attention to gentle cleaning and nutrient support during these periods helps minimize long-term impact. After childbirth, supporting recovery with balanced nutrition and adequate sleep is equally important, as hormonal fluctuations can continue for months and affect gum healing and bone density.

Menopause requires a different approach, focusing on maintaining bone strength and combating dry mouth that often accompanies reduced estrogen. Calcium and vitamin D become even more critical during this stage, as does hydration to support saliva production. Weight-bearing exercise benefits the jawbone as much as the hips and spine, reinforcing the idea that lifestyle habits have oral as well as systemic benefits. Postmenopausal women may also benefit from periodic dental checkups that include bone density assessments of the jaw to catch early changes that could compromise tooth stability.

For men, hormonal changes are more gradual but still relevant. Declines in testosterone over time can influence bone metabolism and indirectly affect gum health through shifts in muscle mass and insulin sensitivity. Supporting metabolic health through diet, movement, and stress reduction offers protective benefits for oral tissues, even in the absence of dramatic hormonal fluctuations.

Daily routines that integrate oral and systemic care create long-term resilience. Balanced meals built around whole foods help maintain steady blood sugar and reduce inflammatory stress on the gums. Hydration supports saliva flow, which is the body's natural buffer against acid erosion and a vital player in remineralization. Consistent movement, whether structured exercise or simply walking, enhances circulation, delivering nutrients and oxygen to gum tissue and supporting detoxification pathways that influence hormone regulation.

Stress management remains a cornerstone of this holistic approach. Cortisol spikes from chronic stress not only disrupt hormonal harmony but also encourage behaviors that harm oral health, such as teeth grinding or neglecting proper hygiene. Small daily practices, like taking mindful pauses before meals or ending the day with deep breathing, gradually retrain the nervous system toward balance. Over time, these habits improve not just mental clarity but also the physical resilience of teeth and gums.

Professional care should be viewed as part of an ongoing partnership rather than a last resort when problems arise. Regular dental visits allow early identification of hormonal effects on oral tissues, from subtle gum recession to changes in bone density visible on X-rays. Collaborative care between dental professionals and physicians becomes especially valuable during major hormonal transitions, ensuring that oral symptoms are not dismissed but understood in the context of broader health patterns.

Sustaining hormonal balance is less about achieving perfection and more about consistency. Small choices made daily—choosing nutrient-dense foods, prioritizing rest, staying hydrated, and practicing mindful stress relief—accumulate into profound long-term benefits. As hormones shift with age, these habits act as stabilizers, buffering the mouth against inflammation, mineral loss, and microbial imbalance. The result is an oral environment capable of withstanding life's inevitable changes, preserving strong teeth, healthy gums, and overall vitality well into later years.

Part IV. Building Your Daily Oral Healing Ritual

Lasting oral health is not achieved through a single treatment or occasional burst of effort but through the rhythms of what you do every day. The mouth responds quickly to both care and neglect, and the habits you repeat—how you breathe, what you eat, the way you clean and protect your teeth—create an ongoing dialogue between your body and its healing systems. This final section is about transforming that dialogue into a ritual, something that not only prevents problems but actively restores balance and supports overall vitality.

Daily oral care often focuses on mechanics: brushing, flossing, perhaps a mouthwash. While these are important, they do not address the deeper influences of diet, stress, sleep, and microbiome balance. True healing rituals integrate these dimensions, weaving oral care into broader routines that nurture the entire body. The mouth cannot be separated from digestion, hormones, or immune function. When these systems work in harmony, gums resist inflammation more easily, enamel recovers from daily acid exposure, and even breath quality reflects inner health.

This approach is not about rigid rules or perfection but about creating consistency. Small, repeatable actions performed at key moments—waking, eating, resting—become anchors that signal safety and renewal to your body. Over time, these rituals shift the baseline: inflammation quiets, mineral balance stabilizes, and the mouth becomes a place of resilience rather than vulnerability.

In the chapters that follow, you will learn how to craft a personalized oral healing routine rooted in both modern science and time-tested natural practices. You will see how nutrition, gentle detox strategies, breathing techniques, and mindful hygiene work together to rebuild balance. Rather than relying on quick fixes or harsh interventions, this ritual cultivates a steady environment in which teeth and gums can strengthen naturally.

The goal is not simply to maintain your current oral health but to elevate it—to give your mouth the conditions to heal and stay healthy for decades to come. By the end of this part, you will have a clear, practical framework to integrate these practices into your life in a way that feels natural and sustainable, empowering you to care for your mouth with the same intention you bring to the rest of your health.

Chapter 10: Designing Your Morning and Evening Routines

A Step-by-Step Daily Regimen for Oral Healing and Maintenance

A healing oral routine begins with understanding that every action you take throughout the day either supports or undermines the health of your teeth and gums. Each moment—morning, meals, nighttime—presents opportunities to create conditions for healing rather than harm. Building a step-by-step daily ritual is less about perfection and more about rhythm: doing the right things consistently so your mouth can restore itself naturally over time.

Morning: Setting the Foundation for the Day

The first minutes after waking shape the oral environment for the entire day. Overnight, saliva production slows and bacteria multiply, which is why many people wake with a coated tongue and a less-than-fresh taste in their mouth. Before eating or drinking anything, begin with a cleansing ritual that resets the mouth's balance.

Rinsing with plain water or a gentle saltwater solution clears away debris and reduces the acidic load that builds overnight. For those who incorporate oil pulling, this is the ideal time: swishing coconut or sesame oil for several minutes helps remove bacterial buildup and primes the mouth for the day ahead. Tongue scraping follows naturally, removing the biofilm on the tongue that contributes to bad breath and restores taste perception.

Brushing comes next, but technique matters more than force. A soft-bristled toothbrush angled toward the gumline, combined with gentle circular motions, effectively removes plaque without damaging enamel or irritating tissues. Choosing a remineralizing toothpaste with fluoride or hydroxyapatite provides added protection against acid wear and supports enamel repair. Flossing, whether with traditional floss or a water flosser, ensures the spaces between teeth—often missed by brushing—stay clean and free of trapped food particles.

Finishing the morning routine with hydration is as important as cleaning. Drinking water stimulates saliva flow, which naturally buffers acids and carries minerals throughout the mouth. A glass of water before coffee or breakfast helps prevent dry mouth and primes digestion, reinforcing the connection between oral and gut health.

Nutrition Throughout the Day

Oral healing is supported not only by what you remove but also by what you provide. Each meal is an opportunity to supply the minerals and vitamins necessary for strong enamel and healthy gums. Foods rich in calcium, phosphorus, vitamin D, and vitamin K2 form the backbone of remineralization, while antioxidants from fresh fruits and vegetables help calm inflammation.

Balanced meals that stabilize blood sugar are equally important. Constant spikes from refined carbohydrates feed harmful bacteria and contribute to acid production, while steady energy from whole foods supports hormonal and immune balance. Adding crunchy vegetables like carrots or celery between meals can help naturally clean teeth and stimulate saliva without relying on processed snacks.

Hydration continues to play a central role. Sipping water regularly throughout the day supports saliva, which remains the body's first defense against acid and bacteria. Herbal teas without added sugar can also soothe tissues and provide beneficial compounds like polyphenols, which have mild antimicrobial effects. Avoiding constant grazing allows the mouth to recover between meals, reducing the time teeth spend in an acidic environment.

Evening care is where the day's cumulative effects are reset and healing is given space to occur. The hours spent sleeping are a period of natural repair, so preparing the mouth properly before rest ensures that this time is used to restore balance rather than allow harmful bacteria to thrive. Brushing thoroughly but gently after the final meal is essential, paying attention not just to tooth surfaces but also the gumline where plaque tends to settle. Flossing or using an interdental cleaner at night becomes even more important than in the morning, as food particles left overnight can quickly turn into acids and biofilm that irritate gums.

A final rinse with water or a mild saltwater solution helps remove residual food particles and neutralize acidity. Those dealing with ongoing gum sensitivity or dryness can benefit from a rinse that includes soothing herbal infusions, like chamomile or aloe, chosen carefully for safety and compatibility with daily use. If dry mouth is an issue, sipping water shortly before bed or using a humidifier in the bedroom can make a noticeable difference in maintaining a protective layer of moisture overnight.

Sleep position can also subtly influence oral health. Breathing through the nose rather than the mouth preserves saliva levels and reduces dryness. People who struggle with mouth breathing may find that addressing nasal congestion, using supportive pillows, or practicing relaxation techniques before bed improves their ability to keep the mouth closed during sleep. Over time, this small shift reduces enamel erosion and gum irritation caused by chronic dryness.

Weekly practices complement the daily routine by targeting areas that benefit from extra care without overwhelming the schedule. These include gentle polishing with baking soda or remineralizing powders to support enamel strength, short oil pulling sessions for those who find them soothing, or focused gum massages to stimulate circulation. These practices do not replace daily brushing and flossing but enhance their effects, especially for individuals rebuilding oral resilience after years of imbalance.

Dietary adjustments also work best when planned over the course of a week rather than obsessing over every meal. Ensuring that several meals each week emphasize mineral-rich foods like leafy greens, grass-fed dairy, or small oily fish provides a steady supply of nutrients that strengthen teeth and bones. Including fermented foods for probiotics and fiber-rich vegetables for prebiotics creates a favorable environment for both oral and gut microbiomes, reinforcing the mouth's natural defenses.

Consistency is what turns these practices into a ritual rather than a checklist. Over time, the body begins to associate certain moments—morning cleansing, evening brushing—with renewal and protection. This rhythm reduces stress around oral care and integrates it seamlessly into daily life. It also prevents the cycle of neglect and overcorrection that often leads to frustration or burnout when trying to improve health habits.

Adapting the regimen to changing needs is part of keeping it sustainable. Illness, travel, hormonal shifts, or life transitions may call for small modifications without abandoning the core principles. The goal is resilience rather than rigidity, trusting that even small, steady efforts contribute to lasting healing. By approaching oral care in this way, you create not only healthier teeth and gums but also a deeper awareness of how the body responds to daily nourishment, rest, and mindful attention. Over months and years, this awareness evolves into a quiet form of mastery—an understanding that your mouth, like the rest of your body, thrives on simple but consistent acts of care performed with intention.

Integrating Herbal Rinses, Oil Pulling, and Natural Brushing

Natural oral care practices have been used for centuries across cultures, often relying on simple ingredients drawn from plants and oils rather than synthetic chemicals. Modern research is beginning to validate many of these approaches, showing that herbal compounds can reduce harmful bacteria, soothe inflamed tissues, and support the balance of the oral microbiome. Integrating these methods into a daily routine can enhance healing and create a more holistic approach to oral care, provided they are used thoughtfully and with a clear understanding of their benefits and limitations.

Herbal Rinses and Their Benefits

Herbal rinses are one of the simplest ways to incorporate natural ingredients into daily oral care. Unlike conventional mouthwashes that often contain alcohol or harsh antiseptics, herbal rinses aim to support the body's natural defenses rather than sterilize the mouth completely. Plants such as chamomile, sage, and calendula are known for their soothing properties and have been traditionally used to calm gum irritation. Others, like clove and myrrh, are naturally antimicrobial and can help reduce the bacterial load that contributes to plaque buildup and bad breath.

Preparing a basic herbal rinse can be as simple as steeping dried herbs in hot water, allowing them to cool, and swishing for thirty to sixty seconds after brushing. For those seeking more convenience, concentrated herbal extracts or tinctures can be diluted in water to create a quick rinse. The key is choosing ingredients that are safe for daily use and avoiding formulas that may irritate sensitive tissues or disrupt the natural pH of the mouth.

While herbal rinses can complement brushing and flossing, they are not a substitute for mechanical plaque removal. Their primary value lies in reducing inflammation, freshening breath, and supporting the overall balance of the oral ecosystem. People recovering from gum irritation or seeking a gentle alternative to strong commercial mouthwashes often find these rinses especially helpful.

The Role of Oil Pulling

Oil pulling, an ancient practice with roots in Ayurveda, involves swishing oil in the mouth for several minutes to support oral detoxification and balance. Traditionally performed with sesame oil, modern variations often use coconut oil due to its pleasant taste and mild antibacterial properties. The process is simple: a spoonful of oil is swished gently around the mouth for ten to fifteen minutes, then spat out and followed by regular brushing.

Studies suggest that oil pulling may reduce levels of harmful bacteria like *Streptococcus mutans* and decrease plaque formation over time. The mechanical action of swishing oil helps loosen debris and coats the teeth and gums, which may contribute to a smoother, cleaner feeling afterward. Additionally, oil's fat-soluble properties allow it to bind with certain toxins and byproducts, potentially reducing oral odor and inflammation.

Consistency matters more than frequency with oil pulling. Performing it a few times per week can still provide benefits without adding unnecessary strain to a daily routine. For many people, combining oil pulling with morning practices like tongue scraping creates a cohesive ritual that feels both cleansing and grounding.

Natural brushing is another area where traditional practices meet modern understanding. Long before commercial toothpaste existed, many cultures used simple powders or pastes made from ground herbs, clays, or mineral salts. These substances provided gentle abrasion to remove plaque while delivering trace minerals and plant compounds that supported gum health. Today, natural brushing can take the form of commercially available tooth powders or homemade blends, but the same principle applies: clean effectively without harsh chemicals or unnecessary additives.

Tooth powders typically include a base of calcium carbonate or clay, which polishes enamel and helps neutralize acids. Herbs such as clove, neem, or peppermint may be added for their antimicrobial and soothing properties, while baking soda provides mild alkalinity. Some blends incorporate xylitol, a naturally occurring sugar alcohol that discourages cavity-causing bacteria without feeding them. The goal is not to strip the mouth of all bacteria but to maintain an environment where beneficial microbes can thrive and harmful species remain in check.

When using natural brushing alternatives, technique remains more important than the ingredients themselves. A soft-bristled toothbrush and gentle circular motions protect gum tissue and enamel regardless of the medium applied. Overly abrasive powders or aggressive brushing can damage teeth, so formulas and habits should be chosen with care. For those who prefer a hybrid approach, alternating between natural powders and conventional toothpaste with fluoride or hydroxyapatite can combine the benefits of both worlds: remineralization alongside gentle plant-based support.

Integrating herbal rinses, oil pulling, and natural brushing into a daily routine works best when viewed as complementary rather than competitive with conventional care. Brushing twice daily and flossing remain the foundation of oral hygiene, with these additional practices layered in for their anti-inflammatory, balancing, and soothing effects. Herbal rinses may be used after brushing to calm sensitive gums, while oil pulling can be scheduled a few mornings each week to reduce plaque and freshen breath. Natural brushing powders may serve as a primary option for some, or as an occasional alternative when seeking variety or avoiding certain additives found in conventional toothpaste.

Safety and consistency are crucial. Not every herbal ingredient suits everyone, and certain essential oils or concentrated extracts can irritate tissues if overused. It is important to ensure that natural powders are finely ground to prevent enamel scratching and that homemade rinses are prepared in clean conditions to avoid contamination. Consulting with a dental professional before making major changes is wise, particularly for individuals managing gum disease, cavities, or sensitivity. Natural methods can enhance healing but should not replace necessary clinical care or corrective treatments.

The deeper value of these practices lies in how they reconnect oral care with mindfulness and intention. Preparing a simple herbal rinse or taking ten quiet minutes to oil pull encourages slowing down and paying attention to how the mouth feels, smells, and functions. Over time, this awareness makes it easier to detect early signs of imbalance—dryness, swelling, or shifts in breath quality—long before they escalate into more serious problems.

By blending ancient wisdom with modern understanding, a holistic regimen emerges that supports both immediate freshness and long-term resilience. These approaches remind us that the mouth is not separate from the body but an integral part of overall well-being. When herbal rinses, oil pulling, and natural brushing are integrated thoughtfully, they transform daily care from a quick task into a restorative ritual, one that nurtures teeth, gums, and the entire system they serve.

Minimalist vs. Advanced Routines: Adapting to Your Lifestyle

Oral healing routines can look very different depending on the season of life you are in, the time you can dedicate to self-care, and the level of structure you are willing to maintain. For some, a minimalist approach is not only sufficient but also more sustainable in the long term. For others, layering advanced practices offers deeper benefits and becomes part of a broader wellness lifestyle. The key is not to adopt the most elaborate routine possible but to match your care to what you can consistently maintain while still supporting your goals for oral and overall health.

When Minimalism Works

A minimalist routine focuses on the essential actions proven to protect teeth and gums: proper brushing, flossing, hydration, and balanced nutrition. For someone with generally healthy teeth, no significant gum issues, and a stable lifestyle, these core practices can maintain resilience without adding unnecessary complexity. Morning and evening brushing with a remineralizing toothpaste, daily flossing, drinking plenty of water, and limiting refined sugars are often enough to keep the oral microbiome in balance.

Minimalism is also valuable during transitional or stressful periods when routines feel overwhelming. New parents, busy professionals, or anyone recovering from illness may find that committing to three or four key actions prevents decline without adding pressure. This approach recognizes that consistency, even in a simplified form, is far more protective than elaborate rituals that are abandoned after a few weeks.

Importantly, minimal does not mean careless. Technique, timing, and awareness still matter. A quick but thorough two-minute brush, mindful flossing, and rinsing with plain water after meals can provide significant protection. Pairing this with nutrient-dense meals rich in calcium, vitamin D, and antioxidants ensures that even a streamlined routine supports both enamel strength and gum health.

The Value of Advanced Routines

An advanced routine goes beyond basic hygiene and intentionally integrates natural practices, targeted nutrition, and lifestyle habits designed to heal and optimize oral health. This approach is particularly valuable for individuals who have active gum inflammation, a history of cavities, or systemic conditions like insulin resistance or hormonal imbalances that affect the mouth. Advanced routines are also appealing to those who view oral care as part of a holistic wellness practice, seeking to harmonize it with other self-care rituals.

These routines often include herbal rinses tailored to soothe or rebalance gums, oil pulling a few times per week, and the use of natural powders or clays to complement traditional toothpaste. Nutritional focus becomes more specific: incorporating foods rich in vitamin K2, omega-3 fatty acids, and probiotics, while carefully avoiding triggers like frequent acidic snacks or drinks. Stress-reducing techniques, posture awareness, and even breathing exercises are included, recognizing their impact on clenching, dry mouth, and gum sensitivity.

The advanced approach also emphasizes timing. Morning routines may involve tongue scraping and gentle rinses to clear overnight buildup before the first meal, while evening care focuses on thorough cleaning and hydration to prepare the mouth for nighttime repair. Weekly or monthly practices, such as gum massages or mineral-rich masks, can provide additional support for those recovering from chronic inflammation or enamel erosion.

Transitioning between minimalist and advanced routines is often fluid rather than fixed. Life circumstances change, and oral care should adjust with them rather than remain rigid. Someone recovering from gum inflammation may start with a more advanced regimen, then scale back once healing stabilizes. Likewise, a person who begins with a simple approach may add elements over time as they gain comfort with new practices and want deeper benefits. This flexibility ensures that oral care remains supportive rather than overwhelming.

A practical way to navigate this transition is to identify a baseline that never changes, regardless of circumstances. For most people, this includes brushing twice daily with proper technique, flossing once daily, staying hydrated, and eating nutrient-rich foods that support mineral balance. From this stable foundation, additional practices such as herbal rinses, oil pulling, or mineral powders can be layered in during periods of heightened focus or specific healing goals.

Maintaining awareness of how your mouth responds is critical when adapting routines. If gums remain tender despite advanced care, it may indicate the need for professional assessment rather than simply adding more steps. On the other hand, if sensitivity decreases and bleeding stops, scaling back to a simpler rhythm can help sustain results without unnecessary effort. This responsive approach turns oral care into an ongoing conversation with the body rather than a checklist imposed regardless of changing needs.

Another consideration is sustainability. Even the most beneficial practices lose impact if they create stress or are abandoned altogether. Minimalist routines work well for those with demanding schedules, travel commitments, or caregiving responsibilities. Advanced routines suit individuals who view oral care as part of a broader wellness lifestyle and are willing to dedicate more time to it. Neither approach is superior; what matters most is alignment with your values, resources, and health goals.

It is also worth recognizing that oral health exists on a continuum with overall wellness. Stress, sleep quality, hormonal fluctuations, and gut balance all influence the mouth. Addressing these factors often creates ripple effects that reduce the need for constant intervention. For example, improving sleep and reducing sugar intake can calm gum inflammation without adding extra rinses or powders. Conversely, ignoring these systemic influences can make even the most advanced routine feel like it is only managing symptoms rather than resolving root causes.

Building a personalized plan means understanding that habits evolve. Some seasons invite a more involved approach with multiple layers of care, while others call for paring back to essentials. The key is consistency in whatever version you choose. Small, steady practices performed daily protect teeth and gums far more effectively than occasional bursts of elaborate care followed by neglect. Over time, this steady rhythm not only maintains oral health but also fosters a sense of trust in your body's ability to heal and stay balanced.

By adapting routines to your lifestyle rather than forcing yourself into an idealized version of oral care, you create a path that is realistic, sustainable, and genuinely supportive. This balanced approach ultimately turns oral health from a burden into a quietly empowering ritual, one that strengthens both the mouth and the broader sense of well-being it reflects.

Chapter 11: Healing Specific Oral Issues Naturally

Supporting Gum Health: Bleeding Gums, Gingivitis, Periodontitis

Healthy gums are the foundation of a strong mouth. They anchor the teeth, protect underlying bone, and form a barrier against bacteria and inflammation. When gum health begins to decline, the earliest signs are often subtle: slight bleeding during brushing, mild swelling, or tenderness along the gumline. Left unaddressed, these early warnings can progress into more serious conditions like gingivitis and periodontitis, which not only threaten teeth but also influence overall health. Understanding how to recognize and respond to these stages is essential for preserving both oral and systemic balance.

Bleeding Gums: The First Signal

Bleeding gums are often dismissed as harmless, especially if they occur only occasionally. In reality, this is one of the body's earliest and clearest signals that something is wrong. Healthy gum tissue does not bleed easily; even gentle brushing should not produce blood. The most common cause of bleeding gums is plaque buildup along the gumline, where bacteria trigger inflammation and make tissues more fragile. This condition, known as gingival inflammation, is reversible if addressed promptly.

Several factors can contribute to bleeding gums beyond poor oral hygiene. Hormonal changes during pregnancy or menstruation, certain medications that affect blood clotting, and nutritional deficiencies in vitamin C or vitamin K can all make gums more prone to bleeding. Chronic stress and systemic conditions like diabetes also increase vulnerability, since they impair immune response and healing capacity. Recognizing these underlying factors is as important as improving daily oral care.

Addressing bleeding gums begins with consistent mechanical cleaning. Gentle but thorough brushing and daily flossing reduce the bacterial load that fuels inflammation. Hydration supports saliva production, which helps neutralize acids and wash away food particles. Nutritionally, prioritizing foods rich in antioxidants and vitamin C aids collagen synthesis and tissue repair. While bleeding may subside within days to weeks of improved care, persistent bleeding requires professional evaluation to rule out deeper gum disease.

Gingivitis: Reversible but Urgent

Gingivitis is the next step on the continuum of gum disease, marked by redness, swelling, and bleeding during brushing or flossing. At this stage, the damage is limited to the soft tissues and has not yet affected the bone supporting the teeth. This makes gingivitis fully reversible with proper care. However, neglecting it allows bacteria and inflammation to penetrate deeper, leading to periodontitis, which is far harder to reverse.

The transition from healthy gums to gingivitis happens gradually, often without pain. Plaque that is not removed within a day or two begins to harden into tartar, which cannot be brushed away and requires professional cleaning. Tartar buildup creates rough surfaces that harbor more bacteria, intensifying inflammation. Over time, gums may start to recede slightly, pockets form between teeth and gums, and bad breath can become more noticeable.

Preventing and reversing gingivitis depends on two key strategies: meticulous daily cleaning at home and timely professional care. Brushing twice daily with attention to the gumline, flossing thoroughly, and using supportive rinses help control bacteria. Professional dental cleanings every three to six months remove tartar and allow for early intervention before damage progresses.

Periodontitis develops when inflammation extends beyond the gum tissue and begins to affect the supporting bone structure. At this stage, the body's immune response to bacteria leads to a cycle of destruction: the gums pull away from the teeth, deep pockets form, and bone begins to erode. Unlike gingivitis, this process is not fully reversible, but it can be halted and managed with proper treatment. Without intervention, teeth may loosen or be lost entirely, and the infection can contribute to systemic problems far beyond the mouth.

Research continues to reveal connections between periodontitis and broader health conditions such as cardiovascular disease, diabetes, and even pregnancy complications. Chronic inflammation in the gums can release inflammatory markers into the bloodstream, influencing the body's immune and metabolic responses. This is why addressing gum health is not merely a matter of preserving teeth; it is a cornerstone of whole-body wellness.

Managing periodontitis requires a partnership between professional care and daily home practices. Deep cleanings, often referred to as scaling and root planing, remove hardened plaque from below the gumline and smooth root surfaces to discourage bacterial buildup. In some cases, local antimicrobial treatments or laser therapy may be recommended to reduce pocket depth and support healing. Consistency with follow-up appointments is critical, as periodontitis tends to flare up if neglected even briefly.

At home, daily habits must become more intentional. Brushing twice a day is not just about surface cleaning but about reaching the gumline with gentle, deliberate strokes to disrupt bacterial colonies. Flossing or interdental cleaning becomes non-negotiable, as plaque between teeth is a major contributor to disease progression. Rinses with mild antimicrobial or herbal formulations can soothe inflamed tissues and reduce bacterial load without disturbing the beneficial microbes that support balance.

Nutrition continues to play a significant role in gum recovery and maintenance. Adequate protein supports tissue repair, while antioxidants from fruits and vegetables reduce oxidative stress that worsens inflammation. Vitamin C and zinc are particularly important for collagen synthesis and immune function, and vitamin D supports bone health, making it crucial for stabilizing teeth affected by bone loss. Hydration, too, supports saliva flow, which helps cleanse the mouth and deliver minerals to both teeth and gums.

Lifestyle factors cannot be overlooked. Smoking is one of the most significant risk factors for periodontitis, impairing blood flow to the gums and reducing the body's ability to heal. Stress management is also essential, as high cortisol levels weaken immune defenses and exacerbate inflammation. Even sleep quality plays a role, since restorative rest allows the body to repair tissues and regulate immune activity effectively.

The most effective gum-healing strategy is not extreme or complicated; it is consistent and attentive. Addressing issues at the first sign of bleeding or tenderness prevents escalation, while regular dental visits catch changes before they become irreversible. For those already managing periodontitis, embracing daily habits that nourish both gums and the broader body creates the best chance of halting progression and preserving function. Over time, these steady efforts transform gum care from reactive treatment into proactive prevention, laying a foundation for lifelong oral and systemic health.

Tooth Sensitivity and Early Remineralization Protocols

Tooth sensitivity can begin subtly, often as a brief twinge when drinking something cold or biting into sweet foods. Over time, this discomfort can intensify, turning everyday meals into a source of anxiety. Sensitivity is one of the earliest warnings that enamel is thinning or gum recession is exposing dentin beneath the surface. Addressing it promptly not only brings relief but also prevents deeper structural problems like cavities or pulp inflammation. Understanding why sensitivity occurs and how remineralization works offers a pathway to both immediate comfort and long-term protection.

Understanding the Mechanisms Behind Sensitivity

The outer layer of each tooth, enamel, is composed primarily of minerals, mainly hydroxyapatite crystals. This structure is incredibly strong but also porous and susceptible to acid attacks from bacteria, food, and even stomach reflux. Beneath the enamel lies dentin, which contains microscopic tubules leading directly to the tooth's nerve center. When enamel wears down or gums recede, these tubules become exposed, allowing hot, cold, or sweet stimuli to reach the nerve endings and trigger pain.

Enamel does not regenerate like bone or skin, but it can be fortified through remineralization. This process relies on replenishing minerals such as calcium and phosphate, often with the help of fluoride or hydroxyapatite to form a stronger crystalline structure. Saliva naturally performs some of this work, but dietary habits, hydration, and pH balance influence how effectively it can protect teeth. Understanding these factors is the first step in designing a protocol that restores balance.

Common Causes That Need to Be Addressed

Several habits contribute to enamel erosion and increased sensitivity. Frequent consumption of acidic foods and drinks, like citrus, soda, or wine, softens enamel and makes it more prone to wear. Aggressive brushing, especially with hard-bristled brushes, can physically erode enamel and cause gum recession over time. Grinding or clenching the teeth, often related to stress, also leads to enamel microfractures and exposes dentin. Even necessary dental procedures such as whitening treatments can temporarily heighten sensitivity by dehydrating enamel and opening dentin tubules.

Systemic factors play a role as well. Reduced saliva flow, whether from medications, dehydration, or mouth breathing, diminishes the mouth's ability to buffer acids and provide essential minerals. Nutritional deficiencies in vitamin D or calcium further weaken enamel and hinder repair. Inflammation from gum disease may expose root surfaces that are not protected by enamel at all, compounding the problem of sensitivity.

Early Intervention Through Remineralization

The goal of remineralization is to restore minerals to weakened enamel before the damage progresses to cavities. This begins by stabilizing the environment: reducing acid exposure, improving oral hygiene, and ensuring adequate saliva production. Avoiding constant snacking and spacing meals allows saliva to naturally neutralize acids and initiate repair.

Fluoride remains one of the most well-researched agents for remineralization. It encourages the formation of fluorapatite, a mineral more resistant to acid than natural hydroxyapatite. For individuals seeking alternatives, bioavailable calcium and phosphate compounds, such as casein phosphopeptide-amorphous calcium phosphate (CPP-ACP) or hydroxyapatite toothpaste, have shown promising results in clinical studies. These materials supply the building blocks needed to fill microscopic weak points in enamel and reduce sensitivity.

Daily practices that support remineralization work best when combined rather than applied in isolation. Gentle brushing twice daily with a toothpaste formulated for sensitive teeth is often the foundation. These pastes either contain fluoride, hydroxyapatite, or compounds that temporarily block dentin tubules, reducing discomfort while the remineralization process takes place. Brushing should always be done with a soft-bristled brush, using circular motions along the gumline to clean effectively without adding further wear to enamel.

Timing can also influence outcomes. Brushing immediately after acidic meals, such as citrus or vinegar-based dishes, can worsen erosion because enamel softens temporarily after acid exposure. Rinsing with water and waiting at least 20 to 30 minutes allows saliva to naturally rebalance pH and harden the enamel surface before brushing. This simple adjustment protects teeth from unnecessary abrasion and enhances the effectiveness of remineralizing agents.

Dietary support is equally crucial. Remineralization depends on a steady supply of calcium, phosphorus, and vitamin D. Leafy greens, dairy or fortified alternatives, nuts, and small fish with bones provide abundant minerals, while vitamin D can be obtained through sunlight exposure or supplementation when necessary. Vitamin K2, found in fermented foods and certain animal products, helps direct calcium to teeth and bones rather than soft tissues, improving structural integrity. Limiting added sugars and processed carbohydrates reduces acid production by bacteria and supports a more balanced oral microbiome.

Hydration plays a quiet but significant role. Saliva is the body's natural remineralizing fluid, carrying calcium and phosphate to weakened enamel. Drinking water throughout the day maintains this flow and helps neutralize acids after eating. Chewing fibrous foods like celery or carrots can further stimulate saliva while mechanically cleaning tooth surfaces. For individuals with chronic dry mouth, sugar-free xylitol gum or lozenges may provide relief and improve protective saliva activity.

In some cases, professional treatments enhance at-home efforts. Dentists may apply concentrated fluoride varnishes, prescribe high-fluoride gels, or recommend products containing calcium-phosphate complexes for intensive remineralization. Sealants can protect exposed dentin in severe sensitivity, while desensitizing treatments temporarily block nerve response during the healing period. These interventions are especially useful when sensitivity stems from enamel defects, early cavities, or gum recession that requires more targeted care than daily routines alone can provide.

Mindful habits outside of oral hygiene also contribute to reduced sensitivity. Managing stress helps minimize clenching or grinding, which accelerates enamel wear and exposes dentin. Wearing a protective night guard can prevent further damage for those with bruxism. Adequate sleep and balanced hormone levels support tissue repair, while reducing inflammatory triggers in the diet benefits both gums and teeth.

Consistency, rather than perfection, determines success with early remineralization protocols. Small improvements compound over time as the oral environment becomes less acidic, better nourished, and more resilient. Even in cases where enamel has thinned, protecting dentin and supporting saliva's natural functions can dramatically reduce sensitivity and prevent further deterioration.

By combining these daily practices with professional guidance when needed, tooth sensitivity becomes not just manageable but often reversible at its earliest stages. This approach empowers individuals to protect their teeth for the long term, transforming a painful warning sign into a catalyst for healthier, stronger enamel and lasting oral comfort.

Addressing Bad Breath and Balancing Oral pH Naturally

Bad breath, or halitosis, is one of the most common oral concerns yet also one of the most misunderstood. It is often treated as a cosmetic issue, something to mask with mints or mouthwash, rather than as a sign of underlying imbalance. In reality, persistent bad breath frequently points to disruptions in the oral microbiome, gum inflammation, or pH changes that allow odor-producing bacteria to thrive. Understanding these root causes and restoring balance naturally can not only freshen breath but also improve overall oral and systemic health.

The Biology Behind Bad Breath

Most cases of bad breath originate in the mouth rather than the stomach or respiratory tract. Sulfur-producing bacteria, particularly those that live on the back of the tongue and between the teeth, break down proteins from food particles and shed cells. This process releases volatile sulfur compounds, which have a distinctly unpleasant odor. While temporary bad breath after eating garlic or onions is normal, chronic halitosis usually reflects a deeper issue: excessive bacterial growth, dry mouth, or gum disease.

pH plays an important role here. A neutral to slightly alkaline oral environment supports beneficial bacteria and keeps harmful species in check. When pH drops due to frequent acid exposure from sugary foods, acidic drinks, or reflux, conditions shift in favor of odor-producing microbes. Acidic environments also weaken enamel and inflame gums, creating a cycle where structural damage and bad breath reinforce each other. Restoring pH balance therefore addresses both odor and oral health at the same time.

Identifying Contributing Factors

Several everyday habits contribute to bad breath. Inadequate tongue cleaning leaves a biofilm on the tongue's surface, a primary source of odor. Skipping flossing allows food particles to decompose between teeth, while chronic dehydration reduces saliva flow, the body's natural cleanser. Certain medications, particularly those for allergies, blood pressure, or depression, can worsen dry mouth and contribute to halitosis.

145

Systemic conditions can also play a role. Uncontrolled blood sugar in diabetes, chronic sinus infections, or gastrointestinal reflux may all produce characteristic odors in the breath. While oral care can help, these situations require medical evaluation to address the root cause. Identifying whether bad breath is purely oral or linked to broader health is an essential first step.

Natural Strategies for Balancing Oral pH

Balancing pH begins with diet and hydration. Frequent snacking on sugary or acidic foods prolongs the time the mouth spends in an acid state. Choosing whole foods, minimizing refined carbohydrates, and spacing meals to allow saliva recovery helps shift the oral environment toward neutral. Drinking water regularly dilutes acids and supports saliva flow, while mineral-rich foods such as leafy greens, nuts, and dairy help buffer acidity and supply the building blocks for remineralization.

Gentle tongue cleaning is one of the most effective yet overlooked habits for reducing bad breath. Using a tongue scraper or the back of a toothbrush, gently remove the coating from the back of the tongue once or twice daily. This simple step can significantly reduce sulfur-producing bacteria and improve overall freshness. Combined with regular brushing and flossing, it forms the core of natural breath management.

Herbal approaches offer additional support by addressing both bacterial balance and inflammation without disrupting the mouth's natural ecosystem. Clove, myrrh, and sage have been traditionally used to calm gum tissues while reducing odor-causing microbes. A simple rinse made by steeping these herbs in hot water can be used after brushing to refresh breath and restore a more neutral pH. Chamomile or green tea rinses provide antioxidant compounds that soothe irritated tissues and may help inhibit the growth of bacteria linked to halitosis.

Essential oils like peppermint or tea tree are sometimes included in natural mouthwashes, but they must be used sparingly and diluted properly to avoid irritating sensitive tissues. Their antimicrobial properties can be beneficial when blended with water or mild carriers, yet overuse may dry the mouth and create rebound effects. The focus should remain on gentle support rather than aggressive sterilization, which often disrupts the balance of good bacteria essential for long-term oral health.

Supporting saliva production is equally vital for fresh breath and balanced pH. Saliva not only washes away food particles but also contains enzymes and minerals that neutralize acids and repair early enamel damage. Staying hydrated is the simplest way to encourage saliva flow, but certain habits can enhance it further. Chewing fibrous vegetables, enjoying sugar-free xylitol gum, or adding a few drops of lemon to water can stimulate the salivary glands without introducing unnecessary sugars or acids. Addressing dry mouth caused by medications or nighttime mouth breathing may require more targeted solutions, such as using a humidifier during sleep or seeking medical guidance for underlying issues.

Lifestyle choices have a cumulative impact on oral pH and breath quality. Smoking, for example, not only dries the mouth but also leaves lingering compounds that contribute to persistent odor and hinder gum healing. Alcohol, particularly in strong commercial mouthwashes, can have a similar drying effect, shifting the oral environment toward acidity and encouraging harmful bacterial overgrowth. Reducing these triggers, or replacing them with supportive alternatives like alcohol-free rinses and herbal infusions, allows the mouth to maintain a healthier equilibrium.

Dietary habits that encourage alkalinity further reinforce these efforts. Meals rich in minerals and antioxidants help buffer acids and provide the raw materials for ongoing enamel repair. Leafy greens, nuts, seeds, and fermented foods supply calcium, magnesium, and beneficial bacteria that contribute to oral and gut balance alike. Limiting highly processed carbohydrates reduces the constant acid challenges that feed odor-producing bacteria. This approach is not about restriction but about creating conditions where the body's natural defenses can function optimally.

Consistency is the key to success. Freshening breath and balancing pH is less about quick fixes and more about small, sustainable actions performed daily. When hydration, mindful nutrition, thorough cleaning, and gentle herbal support become habitual, they create a stable oral environment where bad breath struggles to take hold. Over time, these practices not only eliminate odor but also strengthen enamel, calm gums, and enhance the mouth's ability to protect itself against future imbalance.

By focusing on root causes rather than masking symptoms, these strategies transform bad breath from an embarrassing concern into an early signal of health to be respected and addressed. In restoring pH and nurturing beneficial bacteria, you support not only oral freshness but also a foundation for whole-body vitality, reinforcing the close connection between the state of the mouth and the well-being of the entire body.

Chapter 12: Long-Term Oral Wellness and Prevention

How to Protect Teeth for Decades: Habits That Last

Keeping teeth strong and healthy throughout life is less about expensive interventions and more about consistency with foundational habits. Decay and gum disease do not happen overnight; they develop gradually when small imbalances go unaddressed. The same principle applies to protection. Every deliberate action taken daily, no matter how small, builds toward resilience over the years.

Establishing a Foundation of Daily Care

At its core, lasting oral health depends on mastering the basics. Brushing twice daily with proper technique removes plaque before it hardens into tartar and irritates the gums. The quality of brushing often matters more than the brand of toothpaste used. A soft-bristled brush, gentle circular motions, and attention to the gumline prevent unnecessary wear while thoroughly cleaning surfaces. This approach minimizes enamel erosion and preserves gum tissue over time.

Flossing or using interdental cleaners is equally essential, targeting areas a toothbrush cannot reach. Neglecting these spaces allows bacteria to thrive between teeth, increasing the risk of cavities and gum inflammation. Consistency with interdental cleaning may feel tedious at first, but once it becomes routine, it requires little effort and pays off in long-term protection.

Regular tongue cleaning is another small but impactful habit. The tongue harbors bacteria that contribute to bad breath and biofilm buildup. A simple daily sweep with a tongue scraper or toothbrush can dramatically improve freshness and reduce the microbial load that challenges teeth and gums.

Nutrition as a Protective Force

Diet shapes oral health more than many realize. Sugary snacks and refined carbohydrates fuel acid-producing bacteria that erode enamel, while frequent grazing prevents saliva from neutralizing acids between meals. Shifting toward whole foods with steady meal patterns creates an environment where teeth can recover naturally throughout the day.

Calcium-rich foods like dairy, leafy greens, and almonds supply the minerals needed for enamel strength. Vitamin D from sunlight or fortified foods enhances calcium absorption, while vitamin K2 directs those minerals to the right places in teeth and bones. Phosphorus from nuts, seeds, and lean proteins works alongside calcium to rebuild enamel. Including these nutrients consistently is more effective than occasional supplements or short-term "detoxes."

Hydration also plays a quiet yet critical role. Water supports saliva production, which buffers acids and washes away debris. Choosing water over acidic or sugary drinks preserves the mouth's natural pH and reduces erosion risk. Sipping throughout the day, especially after meals, is one of the simplest ways to support long-term oral health.

Preventing Wear and Tear

Beyond plaque and acids, physical forces threaten teeth over decades. Clenching and grinding, often linked to stress or sleep habits, create microfractures in enamel and accelerate wear. Many people are unaware of this behavior until damage appears as tooth flattening or sensitivity. Stress management, posture awareness, and nighttime mouthguards when needed can protect teeth from this hidden form of erosion.

Chewing habits also influence longevity. Constantly crunching hard foods, ice, or pens can chip or crack enamel, while excessive use of whitening treatments can dry out and weaken teeth. Developing awareness around these seemingly harmless behaviors helps prevent cumulative harm over the years.

Professional care acts as the safety net that complements daily habits. Even with excellent home routines, plaque hardens into tartar over time, and subtle changes in gum health can develop unnoticed. Regular dental visits for cleanings and evaluations allow problems to be caught early when they are easier to reverse. Professional fluoride applications, sealants, or targeted treatments can provide added reinforcement, especially during periods of increased risk such as pregnancy, hormonal changes, or chronic stress.

Consistency with checkups is most effective when they are viewed not as emergency interventions but as part of preventive maintenance. This perspective reduces anxiety and shifts dental care from reactive to proactive. Over years, this mindset helps preserve both oral structures and overall confidence, as routine monitoring prevents minor issues from escalating into major procedures.

Adaptability is another cornerstone of lifelong protection. The habits that serve well in youth may need adjustments as circumstances change. Hormonal shifts, medication side effects, and natural aging all influence saliva flow, gum sensitivity, and bone density. A flexible approach ensures that routines evolve without losing their foundation. For example, someone who experiences dry mouth later in life might increase hydration, incorporate saliva-supportive foods, or switch to toothpaste designed for sensitivity without abandoning their established practices.

Stress management deserves continued attention because chronic tension impacts oral health in multiple ways. Clenching and grinding are the most visible outcomes, but stress also raises cortisol levels, which can weaken immunity and make gums more prone to inflammation. Incorporating daily relaxation practices such as mindful breathing, gentle movement, or time outdoors benefits both mental well-being and oral stability. The mouth reflects the state of the nervous system, and calm habits reduce wear and inflammation over decades.

Long-term success also depends on maintaining a balanced perspective. It is easy to become overwhelmed by conflicting advice or trends promising quick fixes. Focusing on core principles—cleaning thoroughly, nourishing consistently, protecting from acids and mechanical stress—keeps oral health grounded in strategies proven to work across generations. Occasional indulgences, like enjoying sweets or acidic foods, need not derail progress if buffered by strong daily habits and adequate recovery time for saliva and minerals to restore equilibrium.

Technology and new research can enhance but should not replace foundational care. Advances in remineralizing toothpaste, probiotic rinses, or diagnostic tools are valuable, yet their benefits are maximized only when layered onto consistent routines. Awareness of emerging science allows for informed choices, but habits built on simplicity and sustainability remain the backbone of lifelong oral health.

Ultimately, protecting teeth for decades is not about perfection but about accumulation. Every day of proper cleaning, mindful eating, and balanced living strengthens the foundation for the next. Small, consistent actions performed without strain become ingrained over time, transforming oral care from a chore into an effortless part of daily life. When habits evolve naturally and align with the body's needs, teeth remain strong, gums resilient, and the smile a lasting reflection of overall vitality.

Monitoring and Adjusting Your Healing Protocol Over Time

Healing the mouth and maintaining oral balance is not a one-time effort. The body constantly changes in response to diet, stress, aging, and lifestyle, which means a protocol that works well today may need refinement months or years from now. Learning how to monitor progress and make thoughtful adjustments ensures that your efforts remain both effective and sustainable in the long run.

Recognizing the Signs of Progress

The first step in monitoring is knowing what improvement looks like. Healthy gums appear pink and firm, not swollen or red. Bleeding when brushing or flossing should steadily decrease as inflammation resolves. Sensitivity often fades when enamel begins to remineralize and the oral microbiome stabilizes. Breath naturally feels fresher, and discomfort while eating or drinking diminishes.

These positive changes can sometimes be subtle, so paying close attention helps reinforce motivation. Many find it useful to track observations weekly rather than daily. Overly frequent checking can create anxiety, while periodic reflection offers a clearer picture of genuine trends.

Tracking What Needs Adjustment

Not all signs point to healing. If gums remain tender, bleeding persists beyond a few weeks of consistent care, or sensitivity worsens despite remineralizing strategies, these may signal the need for professional evaluation or a shift in approach. Bad breath that lingers even with improved hygiene can indicate deeper gum infection, dry mouth, or digestive issues requiring broader support.

Changes in life circumstances also affect oral health. Increased stress, new medications, or dietary shifts can disrupt the balance you worked to establish. For instance, antihistamines or antidepressants often reduce saliva production, requiring additional hydration and possibly saliva-stimulating strategies. A more demanding work schedule might limit the time you dedicate to oil pulling or herbal rinses, prompting a simplified routine that still covers essentials.

Using Simple Self-Assessments

You do not need complicated tools to monitor oral healing. A mirror and clean fingertips can reveal a great deal about gum tone and texture. Running your tongue along the teeth after meals can help you notice plaque buildup that brushing may have missed. Paying attention to how your mouth feels upon waking provides insight into nighttime dryness, grinding, or the need for adjustments in evening care.

Journaling symptoms and habits can uncover patterns that might otherwise go unnoticed. If sensitivity spikes after certain foods or routines, these details guide smarter modifications. Likewise, documenting improvements reinforces the value of your efforts and builds confidence to continue.

Refinement of your healing protocol often begins with small, deliberate changes rather than complete overhauls. If sensitivity improves but mild gum irritation remains, adjusting focus toward anti-inflammatory strategies, such as herbal rinses or nutrient-dense foods, may create the needed shift. When plaque control is consistent yet breath still feels stale, introducing tongue cleaning or reassessing hydration habits can address overlooked factors without complicating the routine. The goal is to evolve practices in response to feedback from your body, not to chase constant novelty or perfection.

Professional input provides a valuable checkpoint for these adjustments. Regular cleanings and exams reveal progress that may not be visible at home, such as pocket depth reduction or early mineralization of enamel. Dentists can confirm whether a protocol is effectively maintaining gum health or if deeper interventions, like scaling or specialized remineralizing treatments, are warranted. Sharing your daily habits openly allows professionals to tailor recommendations rather than offering generic advice, creating a partnership that respects both natural and clinical approaches.

Balancing structure and flexibility is key to sustainability. A rigid plan can feel overwhelming during stressful seasons of life, while an overly casual approach risks neglecting essential practices. Identifying the non-negotiables—brushing, flossing, hydration—and allowing secondary elements, such as oil pulling or herbal rinses, to rotate based on time and energy preserves consistency without adding pressure. This rhythm acknowledges that healing is a process, not a test of willpower.

Long-term monitoring also benefits from revisiting foundational goals. As gums stabilize and sensitivity decreases, priorities may shift from active healing toward prevention and maintenance. This transition often means fewer specialized interventions and more emphasis on protecting results through steady habits. For example, someone who previously used a mineralizing paste daily might move to using it a few times a week while maintaining nutrient-rich foods and mindful brushing as their primary defense.

Environmental and lifestyle changes should remain part of the conversation. Seasonal shifts in diet, travel routines, or stress levels can subtly affect oral balance. Increased intake of acidic fruits in summer or greater coffee consumption during winter may require extra buffering strategies. Similarly, changes in work or sleep patterns can influence saliva production and immune response. By anticipating these fluctuations rather than reacting to them, you maintain a sense of control over your oral health regardless of circumstances.

A valuable mindset for ongoing adjustment is curiosity rather than judgment. Viewing setbacks—like a return of mild bleeding gums or occasional sensitivity—as information instead of failure fosters resilience. It encourages exploration of root causes rather than reliance on quick fixes. Over time, this perspective transforms oral care from a task to a dialogue with your body, where each symptom or improvement guides the next evolution of your routine.

In the long run, the most successful protocols are those that become part of daily life without constant effort. When habits are refined thoughtfully, guided by both observation and professional insight, they form a foundation strong enough to adapt to change without losing integrity. This adaptability ensures that oral health is not only restored but sustained, allowing teeth and gums to remain resilient through the shifting seasons of life.

When to Seek Professional Care — Integrating Natural and Modern Dentistry

Natural oral healing can do a great deal to restore balance, reduce inflammation, and support remineralization. Yet there are times when professional care is not only helpful but essential. Knowing when to rely on self-care and when to seek expert intervention can prevent minor issues from progressing into painful or irreversible conditions. True oral wellness comes from understanding this balance and creating a relationship between natural strategies and modern dentistry that respects the strengths of both approaches.

Understanding the Threshold for Professional Help

Many people delay dental visits out of fear, cost, or the belief that natural remedies alone will be sufficient. While daily care and supportive nutrition can reverse early signs of gum irritation or mild enamel demineralization, some changes require professional attention. Persistent pain, bleeding that does not resolve after weeks of improved hygiene, visible gum recession, or sensitivity that worsens instead of stabilizing are all signs that deeper intervention may be needed.

Severe toothache, swelling in the face or jaw, or signs of infection such as pus or a bad taste in the mouth indicate urgent care is necessary. These symptoms can point to abscesses or advanced decay that cannot be resolved through home care. Likewise, if a tooth cracks, chips, or becomes loose, prompt evaluation prevents further damage and preserves as much of the natural structure as possible.

The Role of Modern Diagnostics

One of the greatest strengths of modern dentistry lies in its diagnostic tools. X-rays, intraoral cameras, and 3D imaging reveal conditions invisible to the naked eye, such as early bone loss, cavities between teeth, or hidden infections at the root. Even if you prefer to avoid invasive treatments, knowing the exact state of your teeth and gums allows you to make informed decisions about your next steps.

Regular professional assessments also track changes over time. Baseline measurements of gum pockets, bone density, and enamel thickness provide valuable data for adjusting both natural and conventional strategies. This type of monitoring creates a safety net, ensuring that subtle changes are caught early rather than after significant damage has occurred.

Complementing Natural Healing with Professional Support

Integrating professional care does not mean abandoning natural methods. Instead, it allows both to work together. A dentist might clean away hardened tartar that brushing and flossing cannot remove, making it easier for herbal rinses and remineralizing pastes to work effectively at home. Similarly, targeted treatments such as fluoride varnishes or calcium-phosphate sealants can accelerate the body's natural repair processes when used judiciously.

This collaboration also applies to restorative work. If a filling or crown is required, choosing biocompatible materials and ensuring proper follow-up care can minimize disruption to the body's natural balance. Discussing preferences openly with a dentist helps create a plan that respects your desire for minimal intervention while still addressing structural needs.

Choosing the right professional is just as important as recognizing when to seek help. Dentists vary in their training, philosophy, and willingness to integrate natural approaches with modern care. Some are heavily procedure-oriented, focusing primarily on mechanical solutions, while others are open to preventive strategies that align with dietary and lifestyle choices. When searching for a provider, look for someone who respects your desire for minimally invasive care, explains options thoroughly, and is willing to collaborate on a plan that supports long-term healing rather than short-term fixes.

Evaluating a dentist's approach often begins with asking the right questions. Understanding whether they favor conservative treatment, how they view fluoride, or whether they consider the impact of nutrition and systemic health on oral conditions provides insight into whether their philosophy matches your own. Transparency about materials used for fillings, sealants, or crowns can help you avoid substances you prefer to limit, such as certain metals or resins. When both sides share expectations clearly, trust develops, and decisions become easier to make.

Ethical considerations should remain central to any treatment plan. Over-treatment can sometimes occur when financial incentives or fear-based marketing are involved. A trustworthy professional will not rush you into complex procedures but will instead explain the pros and cons, potential alternatives, and timing. They will acknowledge when a watch-and-wait approach is appropriate and when action is needed to prevent harm. This partnership approach encourages you to remain informed and empowered rather than passive.

Integrating natural strategies into professional care requires communication. Sharing details about the herbal rinses, supplements, or dietary changes you use allows the dentist to watch for interactions, evaluate their effectiveness, and guide safe adjustments. In some cases, natural remedies can complement professional treatments, such as using anti-inflammatory herbs alongside scaling procedures to support healing. In others, timing adjustments might be needed to avoid interference, like spacing certain rinses away from fluoride applications so they do not neutralize each other's benefits.

Routine checkups provide an opportunity to reassess your entire oral health strategy. Each visit is a checkpoint to review what has improved, what challenges remain, and whether any underlying conditions are affecting your progress. Life changes such as pregnancy, hormonal shifts, or new medications often call for rebalancing care plans, as these factors can influence gum sensitivity, saliva flow, and susceptibility to cavities. Using dental visits as part of a broader health dialogue ensures that your mouth is treated as an integral part of your overall well-being rather than in isolation.

In emergencies, the value of modern dentistry becomes undeniable. Severe infections, abscesses, and traumatic injuries require immediate intervention that home remedies cannot replace. Prompt treatment can save teeth, prevent systemic complications, and alleviate pain in ways that align with the ultimate goal of preserving natural structure whenever possible. Once stability is restored, natural strategies can then support recovery and prevent recurrence, creating continuity between acute care and long-term wellness.

Ultimately, integrating natural and modern dentistry is about balance and discernment. Neither approach is complete on its own. Natural practices nurture the body's ability to maintain health, while modern tools provide precision when deeper intervention is needed. When these elements work together, you gain the benefits of prevention and innovation without sacrificing your values. Over time, this synergy creates not only stronger teeth and healthier gums but also confidence in your ability to navigate care decisions thoughtfully, adapting to your body's needs at every stage of life.

www.ingramcontent.com/pod-product-compliance
Lightning Source LLC
Chambersburg PA
CBHW070922270326
41927CB00011B/2681